Certified Billing and Coding Specialist (CBCS) Study Guide

EDITION 2.1

AUTHOR
Marilyn Fenichel

REVIEWERS
Rebecca Harmon, MPM, RHIA

Janice O. Campbell, BA HIT, CBCS, CEHRS

Alisa Holliday, CPC, CBCS, CHI

COPY EDITOR
Kelly Von Lunen

GRAPHIC DESIGNERS
Spring Lenox

Randi Janell Hardy

ADDITIONAL CONTRIBUTORS
Derek Prater

Nicole Lobdell

Kaitlyn Mackey

INTELLECTUAL PROPERTY NOTICE

IMPORTANT NOTICE TO THE READER

INTRODUCTION

About $3.7 trillion was spent on health care in the U.S. in 2013. Health care is big business. Qualified billing and coding specialists, like you, will continue to be in demand. Health care practitioners rely on skilled administrative staff for the financial health of their business.

Billing and coding specialists qualify for employment in a variety of settings, including hospitals, clinics, insurance companies, dental offices, and private provider offices, as well as county and government offices. Accepting the challenge to become a part of this growing field requires dedication and a willingness to continually update your skills. Possessing a billing and coding specialist certification will help you support a successful career in this field. This study guide will help you prepare for the National Healthcare Association (NHA) Certified Billing and Coding Specialist (CBCS) certification examination.

In order to sit for the CBCS examination, you must have a high school diploma or a GED and complete a training program. However, you may substitute 1 year of billing and coding experience in lieu of attending a formal training program. With this option, you must provide documentation that you worked as a billing and coding specialist for at least 1 year. If you meet these criteria, you may register for the examination online at www.nhanow.com/billing-coding.aspx.

The CBCS exam consists of 100 multiple-choice questions. If your school is a registered NHA test site, you may be able to take a proctored exam via computer or in paper-pencil format. You also have the option to take the exam via computer at a PSI testing center. For more information about exam eligibility, refer to the Candidate Handbook in the Certifications section of www.nhanow.com.

The key instructional content, or body of each chapter, follows the CBCS test plan. Following the key instructional content, there is a chapter summary that recaps the main points within the chapter and drill questions that assess your knowledge of the chapter subjects. A terms and definitions section at the end of this handbook defines the key words highlighted throughout.

NHA Certified Billing and Coding Specialist (CBCS) Detailed Test Plan based on the 2013 Job Analysis Study; 100 scored items, 20 pretest items

1. Regulatory Compliance   Scored Items: 19

A. Identify appropriate documentation required for release of patient information.

*Foundational Knowledge Enablers:**

1) Verify consent forms are signed and contain all relevant information before the services are rendered.
2) Verify pertinent patient information is released only to authorized individuals.

Critical Thinking Enablers:

3) Compare and contrast informed and implied consent.
4) Compare and contrast use and disclosure.

B. Audit billing against medical documentation to prevent fraud and abuse.

Critical Thinking Enablers:

1) Verify medical documentation with the codes.
2) Compare and contrast fraud and abuse.

C. Identify major laws, regulations, and administrative agencies relevant to medical billing.

Foundational Knowledge Enablers:

1) Adhere to HIPAA, the Stark Law, the Fair Debt Collection Act, and the False Claims Act.
2) Describe the role of the Office of the Inspector General.

2. Claims Processing   Scored Items: 28

A. Apply procedures for transmitting claims to third-party payers.

Foundational Knowledge Enablers:

1) Identify causes of claim transmission errors.
2) Determine the appropriate resubmission method.
3) Differentiate between primary and secondary insurance plans to initially process crossover claims.
4) Compare and contrast "clean" and "dirty" claims.
5) Determine the timely filing limits for claim submission.

Critical Thinking Enablers:

6) Apply knowledge of coordination of benefits.

B. Apply knowledge of the CMS-1500 form to accurately complete the appropriate fields.

Foundational Knowledge Enablers:

1) Identify appropriate placement of NPI numbers.
2) Identify appropriate placement of service codes, DX codes, modifiers, and procedures.
3) Identify appropriate placement of authorization codes.
4) Identify appropriate placement of primary and secondary insurance.

---

*   *Enablers are examples of the task that may appear on the examination, and are not exhaustive lists of the items that may represent the task.*

3. Front-End Duties   Scored Items: 10

   A. Ensure accurate collection of appropriate patient demographic and insurance information.

    Foundational Knowledge Enablers:

     1) Verify changes to demographic and insurance information.

     2) Determine pertinent documents (e.g., insurance cards, identifications, authorizations, referrals) to collect and update.

   B. Verify insurance eligibility to determine benefits.

    Foundational Knowledge Enablers:

     1) Identify how and where to access insurance verification information.

    Critical Thinking Enablers:

     2) Apply appropriate patient insurance rules (e.g., birthday rules, coordination of benefits).

   C. Compare and contrast government and private insurance.

    Foundational Knowledge Enablers:

     1) Identify major types of commercial insurance.

     2) Identify the three government insurance plans.

    Critical Thinking Enablers:

     3) Compare and contrast HMO and PPO plans.

   D. Process appropriate patient authorization and referral forms.

    Critical Thinking Enablers:

     1) Determine when a referral is needed.

     2) Compare and contrast preauthorization, precertification, and predetermination.

   E. Prior to the visit, determine appropriate balances due.

    Foundational Knowledge Enablers:

     1) Calculate the patient's balance due.

     2) Verify the copayment, deductible, and co-insurance percentage.

4. Payment Adjudication   Scored Items: 23

   A. Analyze aging report.

    Critical Thinking Enablers:

     1) Identify which accounts need to be worked first according to office protocol.

     2) Identify reasons for an outstanding balance and appropriate follow-up actions.

   B. Post payment accurately.

    Foundational Knowledge Enablers:

     1) Verify patient name, account number, and date of birth prior to posting.

    Critical Thinking Enablers:

     2) Calculate write-off and adjustment amounts.

C. Interpret remittance advice to determine financial responsibility of patient and insurance company.

Foundational Knowledge Enablers:

1) Determine patient financial responsibility based on remittance advice.

Critical Thinking Enablers:

2) Analyze the remittance advice to determine accurate assignment of benefits.

D. Determine reason for insurance company denial.

Foundational Knowledge Enablers:

1) Interpret denial codes and denial key codes.

Critical Thinking Enablers:

2) Apply definitions of denial codes and denial key codes to determine appropriate resolution.

5. Apply Knowledge of Coding   Scored Items: 20

A. Apply specific coding guidelines and conventions for diagnoses and procedures.

Foundational Knowledge Enablers:

1) Identify the correct code to the highest level of specificity using appropriate ICD, CPT and modifiers, and HCPCS codes.
2) Identify the HCPCS coding convention levels.
3) Identify the structure of ICD coding manuals Volumes 1 and 2.
4) Identify the sections and organization of the CPT coding manual.

Critical Thinking Enablers:

5) Recognize situations where encounter forms should be reviewed with physicians.

B. Abstract the medical documentation by applying knowledge of medical terminology and anatomy and physiology.

Critical Thinking Enablers:

1) Apply knowledge of medical terminology and acronyms.
2) Apply knowledge of anatomy and physiology.

Table of Contents

CHAPTER 1
Regulatory Compliance

OVERVIEW

The coding and reimbursement field is governed by rules and regulations mandated through legislation and overseen by multiple federal agencies. A groundbreaking law, the Health Insurance Portability and Accountability Act (HIPAA) of 1996, was the first uniform standard that included protections for the privacy and security of patient information. It also safeguards against fraud and abuse. Since then, legislation passed as part of the American Recovery and Reinvestment Act (ARRA) was signed into law. A section of the law, the Health Information Technology for Economic and Clinical Health (HITECH) Act, includes changes to HIPAA that relate to privacy. Fittingly, this section is called the Privacy Rule.

These laws lay the foundation for the field. They explain how to receive and manage information so that the patient's confidential medical information is protected. HIPAA, along with a series of other laws, also describes how to prevent fraud and abuse. Other legislation has been passed to further protect Medicare and Medicaid from unlawful practices.

This chapter presents an overview of how to document patient information to maintain a complete, up-to-date clinical record and to protect patient's privacy. Understanding how to protect patient privacy involves understanding what consent forms are and what use and disclosure mean.

The chapter also covers major laws, regulations, and administrative agencies relevant to medical billing. In addition to HIPAA, these include the Stark Law, Fair Debt Collection Practices Act, and False Claims Act. The chapter ends with a discussion of the role of the Office of the Inspector General.

By the end of this chapter, you should be able to answer the following questions.

1. Which of the following accurately describes the difference between informed and implied consent?
   a. Informed consent is required after a procedure, while implied consent is required before a procedure.
   b. Informed consent only refers to electronic documents, while implied consent refers to written and electronic documents.
   c. Informed consent is required in writing after explanation of a procedure, with time to ask questions, while implied consent is assumed.
   d. Informed consent applies to hospitals, while implied consent applies to physicians' offices.
2. What is documentation?
3. Disclosure refers to the way health information is
   a. handled by doctors.
   b. given to an outside person or organization.
   c. stored.
   d. organized.
4. What is the difference between consent and authorization?
5. True or False: Physicians have the option to decide whether to explain privacy rules to their patients.
6. Auditing refers to which of the following?
   a. Writing claims
   b. Signing off on claims
   c. Sending claims to third-party payers
   d. Reviewing claims for accuracy and completeness
7. True or False: Fraud is intentional misrepresentation of information for the purposes of receiving higher payments, while abuse happens unintentionally, often because of poor business practices.
8. Which of the following accurately defines upcoding?
   a. Assigning a code that will deliberately result in a higher payment
   b. Using a shorthand code system
   c. Including more than one procedure in one code
   d. Using multiple codes when a comprehensive code is available
9. The Stark Law states that
   a. debt collection agencies can't use abusive or unfair practices to collect payments.
   b. the government can't be charged for substandard goods or services.
   c. physicians can't refer patients to practitioners with whom they have a financial relationship.
   d. private health information must be kept secure.
10. The Office of the Inspector General is responsible for
    a. protecting health information.
    b. fighting fraud.
    c. helping health care professionals stay compliant with the laws.
    d. disclosing health information.

APPROPRIATE DOCUMENTATION

Documentation is the record of clinical observations and care a patient receives at a health care facility. Documentation is used to communicate relevant patient information among health care professionals. It also serves as the basis of information conveyed to third-party payers, who are responsible for reimbursing providers. Third-party payers include insurance companies, Medicare, and Medicaid.

The documentation must be detailed, current, and accurate. Although information requested can vary from facility to facility, documentation such as the following is usually included.

- Dates of the clinical encounters
- Author of the document
- Patient's medical history and pertinent family history
- Medications the patient is currently taking
- Report of the patient's initial physical examination
- Any allergies, including food and medication allergies
- Physician's diagnostic and therapeutic orders
- Reports and results of every diagnostic and therapeutic procedure performed
  - Laboratory tests performed on blood, urine, and other samples from the patient
  - Pathological examples of tissue samples and tissues or organs removed during surgical procedures
  - Results of imaging procedures, such as ultrasound or MRI

Changes to this list often are based on the facility where an individual is receiving care. For example, the health record kept at a hospital will include the clinical observations of the providers who care for the patient, the patient's discharge summary, and final instructions to the patient upon discharge. In an emergency setting, information about the time and means of arrival at the facility; emergency care given to the patient before and after arrival; medications administered; and a determination of whether the patient will be admitted, discharged, or transferred to another facility is also included.

Informed and Implied Consent

A patient's health record is considered confidential, and there are privacy laws in place to ensure that information is not released without the patient's permission, or consent. Furthermore, providers are required to explain any medical or diagnostic procedures, as well as surgical interventions, and give patients an opportunity to ask questions before any work is done. This is called informed consent. Patients sign documents presented electronically or on paper. Their signature is evidence of their consent.

informed consent. Providers explain medical or diagnostic procedures, surgical interventions, and the benefits and risks involved, giving patients an opportunity to ask questions before medical intervention is provided.

implied consent. A patient presents for treatment, such as extending an arm to allow a venipuncture to be performed.

If a patient voluntarily undergoes treatment, implied consent is assumed. The thinking behind this kind of consent is that it is reasonable to assume that the patient would not agree to a procedure unless he or she understands what it is and what consequences are possible.

It is mostly up to the physician to make sure that the patient understands what the procedure involves, associated risks and complications, and its benefits before the procedure is performed. The patient also should be informed about alternative treatments. Procedures that require the use of anesthesia or experimental drugs, involve surgical manipulation of organs and tissues, or carry a significant risk of complications require written consent. Written consent should be witnessed by at least one person and should be obtained before the service or procedure is conducted. Original or scanned copies should always become part of the patient's health record.

What is the difference between informed and implied consent?

ANSWER: Informed consent refers to the process of explaining any medical or diagnostic procedures, as well as surgical interventions, to patients and giving them the opportunity to ask questions before any work is done. Documents verifying that this has taken place must be signed. If a patient voluntarily undergoes treatment, then consent is assumed. This is called implied consent, and signatures are not required.

Legislation Protecting Patient's Privacy

In 2009, the ARRA was signed into law. A section of the law, the HITECH Act, includes changes to the HIPAA Privacy Rule. This section discusses those changes and how they affect documentation procedures.

To further understand the implications of the Privacy Rule, it is important to know the definitions of the following terms.

Protected Health Information (PHI)

The Privacy Rule has a specific definition for PHI: individually identifiable health information transmitted by electronic media, maintained in any electronic medium, or maintained in any other form or medium (section 160.103). This includes paper forms or documents verifying conversations. To meet the definition of PHI, the information must be held or transmitted by a covered entity or a business associate (BA). Covered entities are any health plan, clearinghouse, or providers. BAs are any individuals, groups, or organizations who are not members of the covered entity's workforce that perform functions or activities on behalf of or for a covered entity. These activities can involve patient health information.

Individually identifiable means the following.

- Documents that either identify the person or provide enough information that the person could be identified

- Information that includes past, present, or future physical or mental health conditions

- Information that includes provision of health care

- Information that includes payment for the provision of health care

clearinghouse. Agency that converts claims into a standardized electronic format, looks for errors, and formats them according to HIPAA and insurance standards.

individually identifiable. Documents that identify the person or provide enough information so that the person could be identified.

Use

The way PHI is handled internally by a covered entity or its business associate.

Disclosure

The way PHI is disseminated from a covered entity or its BA to an outside person or organization. The Privacy Rule applies to PHI requests by covered entities and their BAs.

Minimum Necessary Standard

When disclosing information, providers and other covered entities must limit uses, disclosures, and requests to only the amount needed to accomplish a specific purpose. For example, if information is being disclosed for payment purposes, only what is needed to substantiate a claim should be released.

Notice of Privacy Practices

The legal obligation of providers to explain to patients how their PHI will be used and disclosed. Notice of privacy practices also must explain the patient's rights and the covered entity's legal responsibilities with respect to PHI. Providers who have a direct treatment relationship with an individual must provide this information at the first time of service, either in the physician's office or at a hospital.

de-identified information. Information that does not identify an individual because unique and personal characteristics have been removed.

It is important to note that the Privacy Rule does not protect de-identified information, which is information that does not identify an individual because personal characteristics have been stripped from it.

To ensure that de-identification has been done properly, the Privacy Rule requires the covered entity to do one of the following.

- Strip off certain elements to ensure that the patient's information is impossible to identify.
- Have an expert apply generally accepted statistical and scientific principles and minimize the risk that the information might be used to identify an individual.

Authorizations

The Privacy Rule gives the term authorization specific meaning. Authorization means permission granted by the patient or the patient's representative to release information for reasons other than treatment, payment, or health care operations. In the past, the terms consent and authorizations were used interchangeably, but now consent is used only when the permission is for treatment, payment, or health care operations. Authorizations are always required for use or disclosure of psychotherapy notes.

consent. A patient's permission evidenced by signature.

authorization. Permission granted by the patient or the patient's representative to release information for reasons other than treatment, payment, or health care operations.

Authorization to disclose information applies to the health care facility. It allows the facility to verbally disclose or send health information to other organizations. The patient or the patient's legal representative must sign the authorization, which is kept to document why health information was disclosed.

Authorizations must include the following elements (section 164.508(c)).

- A specific, meaningful description of the information to be used or disclosed
- The name or other specific identification of the person or persons or class of persons authorized to make the requested use or disclosure
- The name or other specific identification of the person or persons of class of persons to whom the covered entity may make the requested use or disclosure

- An expiration date or event that relates to the individual or the purpose of the use or disclosure

- A statement of the individual's right to revoke the authorization in writing and the exception to the right to revoke, with a description of how the individual may revoke

- A statement that information used or disclosed pursuant to the authorization may be subject to redisclosure by the recipient and no longer protected by this rule

- Signature of the individual and the date

- When the authorization is signed by a personal representative of the individual, a description of the representative's authority to act for the individual

To summarize, PHI may not be used or disclosed by a covered entity unless the individual who is the subject of the information authorizes the use or disclosure in writing. There are two instances when the Privacy Rule requires use or disclosure without the individual's authorization.

- When the individual or individual's personal representative requests access to or an accounting of disclosures of the PHI

- When the Department of Health and Human Services (HHS) is conducting an investigation, review, or enforcement action

Under the Privacy Rule, disclosure is permitted without patient authorization under circumstances such as the following.

- When patients have the opportunity to informally agree or object to activities such as being in a patient directory or notifying friends and relatives about their health status.

- When the public health of the community is at risk. For example, if there is an outbreak of tuberculosis in the community, disclosure is permitted to protect the health and safety of the community.

- When legal issues are involved. For example, if an individual has been a victim of abuse, neglect, or domestic violence, disclosure is permitted.

BILLING AUDITS

The previous section introduced documentation, which is a record of a patient's health symptoms, condition, results of the physician's examination, and lab tests. Documentation is presented in a narrative format.

In addition to being used by providers, documentation is also used for billing purposes. The narrative description of the patient's disease or injuries, as well as diagnosis and procedures performed, is translated into a series of codes. These codes are made up of a combination of letters and numbers. The U.S. is in the process of transitioning to a new coding system, which will be described in detail in Chapter 5.

The code sets are a key part of claims, a statement of services and medical conditions submitted by health care providers and facilities. The claim is a record of the medical and surgical services provided to a patient during an episode of care. Accurate claims are submitted to a third-party payer, usually an insurance company, Medicare, or Medicaid. Providers and facilities then receive reimbursement, or payment for services rendered. Reimbursement comes from a third-party payer.

reimbursement. Payment for services rendered from a third-party payer.

Auditing is the review of claims for accuracy and completeness. Many facilities have internal auditing systems to ensure that the claims comply with accepted standards for reimbursement purposes. One of the main things an audit looks for is nonspecific or inaccurate use of diagnosis and procedure codes.

The first step in filling out a claim correctly is knowing how to use the code sets. Under HIPAA, HHS has adopted codes for diagnoses and procedures for all transactions. The adopted code sets for procedures, diagnoses, and drugs are the following.

- HCPCS (ancillary services/procedures)
- CPT-4 (physicians' procedures)
- CDT (dental terminology)
- ICD-10-PCS (hospital inpatient procedure codes)
- ICD-10-CM (diagnosis codes)
- NDC (National Drug Codes)

Chapter 5 will explain these codes and how they should be used. For now, know that understanding codes is part of being compliant, or following established rules, regulations, and guidelines.

The Importance of Being Compliant

Being compliant is an essential part of the job of coding, billing, and reimbursement professionals. It is also necessary to perform at an acceptable skill level. Furthermore, professionals must show integrity in all their decision-making. The AHIMA Standards of Ethical Coding is the place to go for guidelines that professionals in the field need to know.

By not following the guidelines, individuals are at risk for committing fraud and abuse.

Medicare defines fraud as "making false statements of representations of material facts to obtain some benefit or payment for which no entitlement would otherwise exist." In other words, fraud is when something is said that is not true for the purposes of receiving payments. Billing for a service that was not rendered is an example of fraud.

Specific examples of fraud include the following.

- Knowingly billing for services or supplies not provided, including billing Medicare for appointments that the patient failed to keep.
- Knowingly altering claim forms to receive a higher payment. Upcoding is an example of this. Upcoding is when a diagnosis or procedure code is assigned specifically to receive a higher level of payment. Assigning a cough with the code for pneumonia is an example of upcoding.

Another way codes can be misused is through unbundling. Unbundling is the practice of using multiple codes that describe different components of a treatment instead of using the correct single code that describes all steps of the procedure.

auditing. Review of claims for accuracy and completeness.

fraud. Making false statements of representations of material facts to obtain some benefit or payment for which no entitlement would otherwise exist.

upcoding. Assigning a diagnosis or procedure code at a higher level than the documentation supports, such as coding bronchitis as pneumonia.

Abuse refers to practices that, either directly or indirectly, result in unnecessary costs to the Medicare program. Abuse includes any practice that is not consistent with the goals of providing patients with services that are medically necessary, meet professionally recognized standards, and are fairly priced.

Other examples of abuse include the following.

- Charging excessively for services or supplies

- Billing for services that were not medically necessary

- Misusing codes on a claim

As mentioned earlier, conducting audits internally is a way to prevent submitting claims that are either fraudulent or reflect abuse. Numerous laws and regulations are also in place to help professionals submit claims correctly. Several government agencies are charged with monitoring medical billing. The next section explains how these safeguards work together to limit Medicare and Medicaid fraud and abuse.

unbundling. Using multiple codes that describe different components of a treatment instead of using a single code that describes all steps of the procedure.

abuse. Practices that directly or indirectly result in unnecessary costs to the Medicare program.

What is the difference between fraud and abuse?

ANSWER: Fraud is intentionally misrepresenting services rendered for the purpose of receiving a higher payment. Abuse refers to practices that are often done unknowingly as a result of poor business practices, directly or indirectly resulting in unnecessary costs to the program through improper payments. The difference between fraud and abuse is the individual's intent.

LAWS, REGULATIONS, AND ADMINISTERING AGENCIES

Fraud and abuse are serious problems. To minimize their occurrence, a series of laws are in place. These include HIPAA, the Stark Law, the Fair Debt Collection Practices Act, and the False Claims Act. Specific federal agencies play an important role in enforcing these laws.

HIPAA's Role in Protecting Against Fraud and Abuse

In addition to playing a key role in ensuring privacy, HIPAA also has regulations related to fraud and abuse. The key areas targeted by HIPAA are medical necessity (providing appropriate care for a given diagnosis), upcoding, unbundling, and billing for services not provided.

The law also mandated that information about fraud and abuse be compiled into the national Healthcare Integrity and Protection Data Bank (HIPDB). Due to the existence of overlapping data, all HIPDB information will be transitioning to the National Practitioner Data Bank (NPDB). According to HHS, the type of information that must be reported to NPDB includes the following.

- Federal or state licensing and certification actions, including revocation, reprimands, censures, probations, suspensions, and any other loss of license, or the right to apply for or renew a license, whether by voluntary surrender, non-renewability, or otherwise

- Exclusion from participation in federal or state health care programs

- Any other actions or decisions defined in the NPDB regulations

Only federal and state government agencies are required to report such violations. Access to NPDB is limited to those organizations, practitioners, providers, and suppliers.

Final Rule

In January 2013, the Office of Civil Rights (OCR), part of HHS, issued extensive changes to HIPAA. The changes relate to the nature of agreements between covered entities and their business associates, who often assume billing responsibilities. Under the Final Rule, business associates must ensure that PHI remains secure, and they are expected to report any breaches in security.

Compliance with the Final Rule was set for September 22, 2014. The OCR oversees compliance, and has the discretion to resolve violations informally. If necessary, OCR can impose a monetary penalty.

Physician Self-Referral Law (Stark Law)

This law states that physicians are not allowed to refer patients to a practitioner with whom they have a financial relationship. The law also prohibits the referred practitioner from presenting claims to Medicare. The Center for Medicare and Medicaid Services (CMS) has oversight responsibilities of this law.

The services for which referrals cannot be made include the following.

- Clinical laboratory services

- Physical therapy

- Occupational therapy

- Speech and language therapy

- Radiation and imaging services

- Radiation therapy services and supplies

- Durable medical equipment and supplies

- Parenteral and enteral nutrients, equipment, and supplies

- Prosthetics, orthotics, and prosthetic devices and supplies

- Home health services

- Outpatient prescription drugs

- Inpatient and outpatient hospital services

Fair Debt Collection Practices Act (FDCPA)

This law says that debt collectors, including collection agencies, lawyers, or companies who buy unpaid debts, cannot use unfair or abusive practices to collect payments. Medical bills are one of the debts protected by this law. The Federal Trade Commission is responsible for enforcing FDCPA.

---

business associate (BA). Individuals, groups, or organizations who are not members of a covered entity's workforce that perform functions or activities on behalf of or for a covered entity.

False Claims Act

The False Claims Act protects the government from being overcharged for services provided or sold, or substandard goods or services. Penalties, which include fines and damages up to three times the amount sustained by the government, are associated with any physician who knowingly submits a false or fraudulent claim. "Knowing" includes doing this in "deliberate ignorance" or with "reckless disregard of the truth related to the claim." For example, a physician who submits a claim to Medicare for services that she knows were not provided is in violation of the False Claims Act.

Role of the Office of the Inspector General (OIG)

HIPAA established a comprehensive program to combat fraud called the Health Care Fraud and Abuse Control (HCFAC) Program. Housed in the OIG, the program is run jointly by the Department of Justice and HHS. The OIG protects Medicare and other HHS programs from fraud and abuse by conducting audits, investigations, and inspections to answer formal complaints.

The OIG has the authority to exclude individuals and entities who have engaged in fraud and abuse from participating in Medicare, Medicaid, and other federal health care programs. The office also can impose penalties on offenders. The OIG keeps an office List of Excluded Individuals/Entities (LEIE).

In 2009, the Department of Justice and HHS established the Health Care Fraud Prevention and Enforcement Action Team (HEAT). The purpose of HEAT is to strengthen efforts to fight fraud and invest in new technologies to prevent fraud and abuse. The website www.stopmedicarefraud.gov provides information about how to identify fraud and report it.

What is the main job of the Office of the Inspector General?

ANSWER: The Office of the Inspector General protects Medicare and other HHS programs from fraud and abuse by conducting audits, investigations, and inspections.

SUMMARY

This chapter covered the following topics.

- What complete documentation should include

- Why accurate documentation is important and what it is used for

- The difference between informed and implied consent

- The difference between use and disclosure

- The difference between fraud and abuse

- Laws, regulations, and agencies that protect against fraud and abuse

Understanding these key topics lays the foundation for claims processing and the correct use of certain codes. These topics will be covered in Chapter 2.

CHAPTER 1 DRILL QUESTIONS

Appropriate Documentation

1. Which of the following accurately describes the difference between informed and implied consent?

   a. Informed consent is required after a procedure, while implied consent is required before a procedure.

   b. Informed consent only refers to electronic documents, while implied consent refers to written and electronic documents.

   c. Informed consent is required in writing after explanation of a procedure, with time to ask questions, while implied consent is assumed.

   d. Informed consent applies to hospitals, while implied consent applies to physicians' offices.

2. What is documentation?

3. Disclosure refers to the way health information is

   a. handled by doctors.

   b. given to an outside person or organization.

   c. stored.

   d. organized.

4. What is the difference between consent and authorization?

5. True or False: Physicians have the option to decide whether to explain privacy rules to their patients.

Billing Audits

6. Auditing refers to which of the following?

   a. Writing claims

   b. Signing off on claims

   c. Sending claims to third-party payers

   d. Reviewing claims for accuracy and completeness

7. True or False: Fraud is intentional misrepresentation of information for the purposes of receiving higher payments, while abuse happens unintentionally, often because of poor business practices.

Laws, Regulations, and Administering Agencies

8. Which of the following accurately defines upcoding?

    a. Assigning a code that will deliberately result in a higher payment

    b. Using a shorthand code system

    c. Including more than one procedure in one code

    d. Using multiple codes when a comprehensive code is available

9. The Stark Law states that

    a. debt collection agencies can't use abusive or unfair practices to collect payments.

    b. the government can't be charged for substandard goods or services.

    c. physicians can't refer patients to practitioners with whom they have a financial relationship.

    d. private health information must be kept secure.

10. The Office of the Inspector General is responsible for

    a. protecting health information.

    b. fighting fraud.

    c. helping health care professionals stay compliant with the laws.

    d. disclosing health information.

CHAPTER 1 DRILL ANSWERS

1. **A.** *Incorrect* Informed consent is given before, not after, a procedure.

   B. *Incorrect* Informed consent may be documented electronically or on paper. Implied consent is not documented.

   C. *Correct* This is the correct distinction between informed consent, which requires the patient's signature, and implied consent.

   D. *Incorrect* Whether consent is informed or implied is not based on the setting.

2. Documentation is a complete, accurate, up-to-date record of the care a patient receives at a health care facility.

3. **A.** *Incorrect* Health information can be disclosed by people other than doctors.

   B. *Correct* Disclosure refers to the dissemination of personal health information, which is covered by the HIPAA Privacy Rule.

   C. *Incorrect* Disclosure does not refer to the manner in which health information is stored.

   D. *Incorrect* Disclosure does not refer to the manner in which health information is organized.

4. Authorization is permission granted by the patient or the patient's representative to release information for reasons other than treatment, payment, or health care operations. Consent is used only when the permission is for treatment, payment, or health care operations.

5. False. Physicians are legally obligated to explain privacy rules to their patients.

6. **A.** *Incorrect* Auditing is performed after claims have been written.

   B. *Incorrect* An audit may be performed prior to signing off on a claim, but not every audit would lead to signing off on a given claim.

   C. *Incorrect* Auditing does not refer to the process of sending claims to third-party payers.

   D. *Correct* Many facilities have internal auditing systems to review claims for accuracy and completeness. One of the main things an audit looks for is nonspecific or inaccurate use of diagnosis and procedure codes.

7. True. An example of fraud is knowingly billing for services or supplies that were not provided. Abuse includes any practice that is not consistent with the goals of providing patients with services that are medically necessary, meet professionally recognized standards, and are fairly priced.

8. **A.** *Correct* Assigning a cough with the code for pneumonia is an example of upcoding, and it is fraud.

   B. *Incorrect* Using shorthand is not specific to upcoding.

   C. *Incorrect* This refers to bundling, which is appropriate when a single code describes all steps for a given procedure.

   D. *Incorrect* Unbundling, which is the practice of using multiple codes to describe components of a procedure rather than a single, overarching code, is inappropriate.

9. **A.** *Incorrect* This is covered by the Fair Debt Collection Practices Act.

   B. *Incorrect* This is covered by the False Claims Act.

   C. *Correct* Also referred to as the Physician Self-Referral Law, the Stark Law also prohibits the referred practitioner from presenting claims to Medicare.

   D. *Incorrect* This is covered by the HIPAA Privacy Rule.

10. **A.** *Incorrect* This is not among the OIG's mandates.

    B. *Correct* HIPAA established a comprehensive program to combat fraud called the Health Care Fraud and Abuse Control (HCFAC) Program, which is run by the OIG.

    C. *Incorrect* This is not among the OIG's mandates.

    D. *Incorrect* This is not among the OIG's mandates.

CHAPTER 2
Claims Processing

OVERVIEW

Chapter 1 explained what documentation is and why it is important; discussed key elements of documentation, including consent forms and authorizations; and explained the laws in place to prevent fraud and abuse.

This chapter turns to another important topic: how to submit claims for reimbursement that are clear and accurate. Claims are important because they contain the information third-party payers (Medicare, Medicaid, and insurance companies) need to reimburse providers for their services. If the claims are not filled out and submitted correctly, providers will not be paid.

Medicare has a specific form that providers must fill out, the CMS-1500. The second part of the chapter explains how to fill out this form correctly. That includes what information needs to go in what field, what specific codes need to be used, and where they should go. When filling out the CMS-1500, it is also important to know what an NPI number is, where that belongs on the form, and the difference between primary and secondary insurance.

By the end of this chapter, you should be able to answer the following questions.

1. What is a claim?

2. Identify two items of information that need to be on a claim.

3. Which of the following describes a clean claim?

   a. All the data elements are completed.

   b. All the data elements are written on a white piece of paper.

   c. Almost all the data elements are right.

   d. All the necessary data elements are completed.

4. True or False: In 2012, the Administration Simplification Compliance Act (ASCA), part of HIPAA, mandated that health care claims be submitted electronically, with some exceptions.

5. The primary insurance plan does which of the following?

   a. Pays for everything

   b. Pays first

   c. Pays second

   d. Has the option of paying first or second

6. What is an NPI number? Where does it go on CMS-1500?

7. True or False: Misspelling a patient's name is a common processing error.

8. True or False: You are allowed to use both six- and eight-digits for the date on one claim.

9. Describe when Medicare is the secondary insurance for a patient.

10. By signing block 12 on the CMS-1500 form, a patient is doing which of the following?

    a. Authorizing the release of funds to a provider

    b. Authorizing the provider to perform a procedure

    c. Authorizing the release of medical information needed to process a claim

    d. Authorizing hospice care

Medicare. Federally funded health insurance provided to people age 65 or older, people younger than 65 who have certain disabilities, and people of all ages with end-stage kidney disease. Funded and administered at the national level.

Medicaid. A government-based health insurance option that pays for medical assistance for individuals who have low incomes and limited financial resources. Funded at the state and national level. Administered at the state level.

TRANSMITTING CLAIMS

Information on a Claim

Claims are a complete record of the services provided by the health care professional, along with appropriate insurance information. Table 2.1 identifies the information needed on a correctly filled-out claim.

TABLE 2.1 *Essential Information on a Claim*

INFORMATION	DESCRIPTION
Patient name	Patient's name should be consistent across all documents.
Patient's health record number (used on the UB-1450)	The provider uses this number to identify the patient.
Patient's account number	Identifies specific episode of care, date of service, or hospitalization.
Patient's demographic information	Date of birth, sex, marital status, address, telephone number, relationship to subscriber, and circumstances of condition (such as related to an automobile accident or a pre-existing condition.
Subscriber: member, policyholder, certificate holder, or insured name	Purchaser of the insurance or the member of group for which an employer or association as purchased insurance.
Subscriber (member) number	Unique code used to identify the subscriber's policy.
Group or plan number	Unique code used to identify a set of benefits of one group of type of plan.
Prior approval number (pre-certification or preauthorization number, if applicable)	Number indicating that the insurance company has been notified and has approved the services before they were rendered.
Provider name	Name of hospital, physician, or other entity that provided services.
National provider identifier (NPI)	Unique 10-digit code for providers required by the Health Insurance Portability and Accountability Act (HIPAA) of 1996.
Provider's address and telephone number	Address and telephone number of entity that provided services and will be reimbursed by the claim.
Date(s) of service	Date when the service was provided.
Diagnosis code	International Classification of Diseases code.
Procedure code	ICD-10-CM, Current Procedural Terminology code, or the Healthcare Common Procedures Coding System that represents the procedure or service provided.
Revenue code (used on the UB-1450)	Four-digit code that identifies specific accommodation, ancillary service, or billing calculation related to the services on the bill. Indicates the type of service performed, where the service was performed, and provides a summary of other services and supplies used for treatment.
Itemized charges for services	Detailed list of each service and its cost.
Number of services or duration of time	Details related to number of services or length of time service was provided.
Secondary or other insurance information	Another entity that may be responsible to reimburse the provider for the services rendered, such as automobile insurance or workers' compensation.

Source: Principles of Healthcare Reimbursement, Fourth Edition. pp. 75.

Procedures for Transmitting Claims

Transmitting claims involves sending required information (see Table 2.1) to third-party payers for reimbursement. In most instances, providers file insurance claims to insurance companies or government-sponsored health care insurance programs such as Medicare. The submission process is similar for both types of insurance.

In 2012, the Administration Simplification Compliance Act (ASCA), part of HIPAA, mandated that health care claims be submitted electronically. The exception is that paper claims may be sent to clearinghouses, which then convert the claims into a standardized electronic format. Clearinghouses also look for errors and format them according to HIPAA and insurance standards. Because providers have so much data to transmit, most use clearinghouses with the hope that the number of submission errors will be reduced.

For Medicare, the transaction standard is the Accredited Standards Committee (ASC) X12N version of 5010. The electronic format for facilities is 837-I and 837-P for professionals. These electronic formats correspond to the paper formats of the Uniform Bill 2004 (CMS 1450 Claim Form or UB-04) and the Centers for Medicare and Medicaid Services (CMS-1500 Claim Form, 1500, or CMS-1500). If facilities have a waiver of the ASCA requirements, they should use these paper formats.

When filing claims for Medicare, it is necessary to meet the timely filing requirement. Claims must be received within 1 calendar year of the claim's date of service. If the claim is filed after this timeframe, it will be rejected without an opportunity for an appeal.

For claims that cover a span of several dates, timeliness is determined according to these guidelines.

- For institutional claims, the "Through" date is used to determine the date of service.

- For professional claims, the "From" data is used to determine the date of service.

Exceptions to this requirement include the following.

- An administrative error or misrepresentation on the part of the individual filing the claim

- Retroactive Medicare entitlement

- Retroactive Medicare entitlement involving state Medicaid agencies and beneficiaries eligible for both benefits

- Retroactive disenrollment from a Medicare Advantage Plan or a Program of All-Inclusive Care for the Elderly

The transfer of electronic information, such as health claims, in a standard format is called electronic data interchange (EDI). EDI was put in place because many industries believed that this approach would be the most effective and cost-efficient way to transmit information among multiple partners or covered entities. It has reduced handling and processing time, as well as minimized the risk of lost paper documents. Overall, EDI can reduce the burden on administrative staff, lower operating costs, and improve overall data quality for simplification.

timely filing requirement.
Within 1 calendar year of a claim's date of service.

electronic data interchange (EDI). The transfer of electronic information in a standard format.

Coordination of Benefits

Some patients have more than one insurance policy. For example, they might have Medicare and a health insurance plan through their employer. In those instances, it is important to determine which insurance plan is primary and which is secondary. Coordination of benefits rules makes this determination. The primary insurance pays first, up to the limits of its coverage. If there are costs that the primary insurance didn't cover, the bill goes to the secondary insurance. The secondary insurance, which can be Medicare, might not pay all the costs. If the employer health insurance is the secondary plan, it can be necessary to enroll in Medicare Part B before the insurance plan will pay.

coordination of benefits rules. Determines which insurance plan is primary and which is secondary.

If the insurance company is the primary insurance and does not pay within 120 days, the provider is allowed to bill Medicare. Medicare can make a conditional payment, which is then recovered after the primary insurance pays.

conditional payment. Medicare payment that is recovered after primary insurance pays.

Crossover claims refer to claims submitted by people covered by a primary and secondary insurance plan, such as Medicare and Medicaid. In this example, Medicare receives the bill first, applies a deductible/coinsurance or copay amount, and then automatically forwards it to Medicaid. Providers no longer have to bill Medicaid separately for the Medicare deductible, coinsurance, or copay amounts.

crossover claim. Claim submitted by people covered by a primary and secondary insurance plan.

The same process applies to Medicare and another secondary insurance plan. After the secondary insurance plan signs a coordination of benefits agreement, there is automatic crossover between the primary and secondary insurance.

What is the difference between primary and secondary insurance?

ANSWER: The primary insurance pays first, up to the limit of its coverage. If the primary insurance did not cover all the charges, the bill that is still outstanding is sent to the secondary insurance. The secondary insurance might not pay all the costs.

Causes of Claim Transmission Errors

Even with EDI, both providers and payers still make mistakes. When submitting claims, the following errors are the most common.

- Differences in a patient's name or its spelling, such as a nickname or a hyphenated last name

- Missing or invalid patient identification number

- Missing or invalid patient information, such as sex, date of birth, or Social Security number

- Missing or invalid subscriber (member) name

- Missing or invalid certificate or group number

- Lack of authorization or referral number

- Failure to check the box for assignment of benefits (contract in which the provider directly bills the payer and accepts the allowable charge), or the amount the insurer will accept, as full payment, minus patient's out of pocket cost

- Invalid dates of services

- Missing or invalid modifiers

- Missing or invalid provider information, such as tax identification number or NPI number

- Incorrect place of service

The American Medical Association (AMA) conducts a survey each year to find out how accurately payers reimburse providers. Based on 2011 results, the average claims processing error rate was 19.3%, an increase of 2%, or $3.6 million, over the previous year. These errors added $1.5 billion in unnecessary administrative costs to the health care system. The AMA estimates that $17 billion could be saved if payment errors were drastically reduced or eliminated.

Clean and Dirty Claims

Clean claims are accurate and complete. They have all the information needed for processing, which is done in a timely fashion. Dirty claims are those that are inaccurate, incomplete, or contain other errors, like those listed under "Causes of Claim Transmission Errors." Dirty claims are delayed, often because they are sent back to the provider for correction and resubmission or undergo manual processing by the third-party payer's office.

Name two causes of claim transmission errors.

ANSWER: Missing or invalid patient identification number and lack of authorization or referral number are two causes of claim transmission errors.

Claims Processing

Medicare Parts A and B claims from hospitals, physicians, and other providers are processed by Medicare Administrative Contractors (MACs). Following submission of the claim, the billing professional who sent in the claim will receive a remittance advice (RA). The RA reflects any changes made to the original billing. Adjustments usually fall into one of the following categories.

- Denied claim

- Zero payment

- Partial payment

- Reduced payment

- Penalty applied

- Additional payment

- Supplemental payment

If there are errors on the claim, it must be resubmitted within the timely filing requirement (within 1 calendar year of the date the claim was returned). Unless the claim has been returned because it cannot be processed, an appeal may be filed. This also must be done according to the timely filing requirement.

If the claim was returned because of a clerical error, it is possible to request a reopening to fix the error. This process is different from an appeal. It, too, must be done according to the timely filing requirement.

assignment of benefits. Contract in which the provider directly bills the payer and accepts the allowable charge.

allowable charge. The amount an insurer will accept as full payment, minus applicable cost sharing.

clean claim. Claim that is accurate and complete. They have all the information needed for processing, which is done in a timely fashion.

dirty claim. Claim that is inaccurate, incomplete, or contains other errors.

Medicare Administrative Contractor (MAC). Processes Medicare Parts A and B claims from hospitals, physicians, and other providers.

remittance advice (RA). The report sent from the third-party payer to the provider that reflects any changes made to the original billing.

CMS-1500 FORM

Although the ASCA requires that claims to Medicare be transmitted electronically, if a provider uses a clearinghouse to submit claims, the draft may be completed on paper and converted to 837 for processing. If that is the case, the correct form to use is CMS-1500, which has been revised by the National Uniform Claim Committee (NUCC). Any new version of the form must be approved by the White House Office of Management and Budget (OMB). The revised form is version 02/12, OMB control number 0938-1197.

It is very important to fill out the form correctly. The following section explains what information (referred to as blocks) needs to go in each field.

Member Information

Fields 1 through 13 focus on basic information about the patient, the insured (if that person is not the patient), and if the patient has two insurance plans, determining which is primary and which is secondary (Block 11). This information must be entered exactly as specified.

EXAMPLE 2.1 *CMS-1500 Form*

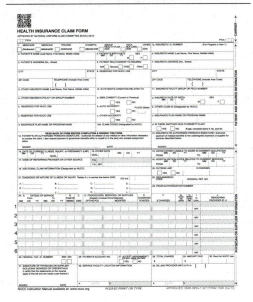

Source: National Uniform Claim Committee

EXAMPLE 2.2 *CMS-1500 Form Blocks 1-8*

1. MEDICARE (Medicare#)	MEDICAID (Medicaid#)	TRICARE (ID#/DoD#)	CHAMPVA (Member ID#)	GROUP HEALTH PLAN (ID#)	FECA BLK LUNG (ID#)	OTHER (ID#)	1a. INSURED'S I.D. NUMBER (For Program in Item 1)
2. PATIENT'S NAME (Last Name, First Name, Middle Initial)			3. PATIENT'S BIRTH DATE MM DD YY	SEX M F			4. INSURED'S NAME (Last Name, First Name, Middle Initial)
5. PATIENT'S ADDRESS (No., Street)			6. PATIENT RELATIONSHIP TO INSURED Self Spouse Child Other				7. INSURED'S ADDRESS (No., Street)
CITY		STATE	8. RESERVED FOR NUCC USE				CITY / STATE
ZIP CODE	TELEPHONE (Include Area Code) ( )						ZIP CODE / TELEPHONE (Include Area Code) ( )
9. OTHER INSURED'S NAME (Last Name, First Name, Middle Initial)			10. IS PATIENT'S CONDITION RELATED TO:				11. INSURED'S POLICY GROUP OR FECA NUMBER

Source: National Uniform Claim Committee

BLOCK 1   Check the box indicating what kind of insurance is applicable, such as Medicare.

BLOCK 1A   The patient's *Medicare Health Insurance Claim Number (HICN)*. This number must be recorded whether Medicare is the primary or secondary payer.

BLOCK 2   The patient's first name, middle initial (if any), and last name, as shown on the patient's Medicare card.

BLOCK 3   The patient's eight-digit birth date (recorded as MM|DD|CCYY) and sex. For example: September 28, 1990, would be recorded: 09|28|1990.

BLOCK 4   If there is an insurance primary to Medicare, obtained through the patient's or spouse's place of work or through any other source, list the name of the insured here. If the patient and the insured are the same, write SAME. If Medicare is primary, leave this field blank.

BLOCK 5   The patient's mailing address and telephone number. Put the mailing address on the first line, the city and state on the second line, and the ZIP code and phone number on the third line.

BLOCK 6   Check the appropriate box to patient's relationship to the insured.

BLOCK 7   Enter the insured's address and phone number. If the insured is the same as the patient, write SAME. Complete this block only after blocks 4, 6, and 11 have been completed.

BLOCK 8   Leave blank.

EXAMPLE 2.3   *CMS-1500 Form Blocks 9-13*

Source: National Uniform Claim Committee

BLOCK 9   Write the last name, first name, and middle initial (if any) of the Medigap enrollee if it is a different person from the one listed in Block 2. Otherwise, write SAME. If no Medigap benefits are assigned, leave blank.

BLOCK 9A   Enter the policy and group number of the Medigap insured preceded by MEDIGAP, MG, or MGAP.

BLOCK 9B   Leave blank.

BLOCK 9C   Leave blank.

BLOCK 9D   Write in the Coordination of Benefits Agreement Medigap-based identifier.

BLOCKS 10A-C   Check "Yes" or "No" to indicate whether employment, auto liability, or other accident involvement applies to one or more of the services listed in block 24. A "yes" answer indicates there might be other insurance primary to Medicare.

BLOCK 11   This is an important field. This is the place to indicate that a good faith effort has been made to determine whether Medicare is the primary insurance. Information about insurance primary to Medicare should be listed in blocks 11a-11c.

Instances where Medicare is the secondary insurance include the following.

- Group Health Plan Coverage
    - Working aged
    - Disability (large group health plan)
    - End-stage kidney disease
- No fault and/or other liability
- Work-related Illness/Injury
    - Workers' compensation
    - Black lung
    - Veterans' benefits

BLOCK 11A   This is where the insured's birth date goes. Enter the sex as well if it is different from Block 3.

BLOCK 11B   For insurance primary to Medicare, enter employer's name, if applicable. If there is a change in the insured's insurance status (e.g., retired), enter either a 6-digit (MM|DD|YY) or 8-digit (MM|DD|CCYY) retirement date preceded by the word "RETIRED." For Tricare and CHAMPVA, enter the sponsor's branch of service, using abbreviations (e.g., United States Navy = USN). For commercial claims, check for payer-specific instructions.

BLOCK 11C   Enter the nine-digit payer ID number of the primary insurer. If there is no payer ID, then write in the primary payer's program or plan name. If the Explanation of Benefits (EOB) does not include the claim's processing address, then write it in.

BLOCK 11D   For Medicare, leave blank. For all other payers, enter an 'x' in the correct box, if appropriate. If marked "YES," complete items 9, 9a, and 9d.

Why is block 11 important?

ANSWER: This is the place to indicate that a good faith effort has been made to determine which is the primary insurance and which is secondary.

BLOCK 12   This is an important field where the patient or an authorized person signs to authorize the release of medical information. The field must be dated and entered as a six- or eight-digit date. A signature on file or a computer-generated signature can also be used. The patient's signature authorizes release of information necessary to process the claim.

BLOCK 13   This signature authorizes payment of benefits to the physician or supplier. A signature on file is acceptable here.

---

explanation of benefits (EOB).
Describes the services rendered, payment covered, and benefit limits and denials.

Rendering Provider

These fields (14 through 33) include information about the providers, services rendered, diagnoses made, procedures performed, and modifiers needs. Each field is described below.

EXAMPLE 2.4 *CMS-1500 Form Blocks 14-18*

14. DATE OF CURRENT ILLNESS, INJURY, or PREGNANCY (LMP) MM DD YY QUAL.	15. OTHER DATE QUAL.	MM DD YY	16. DATES PATIENT UNABLE TO WORK IN CURRENT OCCUPATION MM DD YY MM DD YY FROM TO
17. NAME OF REFERRING PROVIDER OR OTHER SOURCE	17a.		18. HOSPITALIZATION DATES RELATED TO CURRENT SERVICES MM DD YY MM DD YY
	17b. NPI		FROM TO
19. ADDITIONAL CLAIM INFORMATION (Designated by NUCC)			20. OUTSIDE LAB? $ CHARGES

Source: National Uniform Claim Committee

BLOCK 14 For Medicare, for the current illness, injury, or pregnancy, enter either an 8-digit (MM|DD|CCYY) or 6-digit (MM|DD|YY) date. For chiropractic services, enter the date of the initiation of the course of treatment and enter the date of x-ray (if used to demonstrate subluxation) in item 19. Medicare does not use qualifiers.

For commercial claims: Enter the date of the first date of the present illness, injury, or pregnancy. For pregnancy, use the date of the last menstrual period (LMP) as the first date. Enter the applicable qualifier to identify which date is being reported (e.g., 431 Onset of Current Symptoms or Illness, 484 Last Menstrual Period).

BLOCK 15 For Medicare, leave blank (not required). For all other carriers, check for payer-specific instructions. When required, enter another date related to the patient's condition or treatment and the applicable qualifier to identify which date is being reported.

BLOCK 16 Dates patient is unable to work in his current occupation. This is required if the patient is eligible for disability or workers' compensation benefits. To fill out this field, enter the "From" and "To" dates as follows: MMDDYY (051512) or MMDDCCYY (05152012).

BLOCK 17 This is where the name of the referring or ordering physician goes. If Medicare requires that a supervising physician be listed, put that name here. If a claim involves more than one referring, ordering, or supervising physician, a separate claim must be submitted for each. Table 2.2 shows the qualifiers that should be used for each kind of provider.

TABLE 2.2 *Qualifiers for Different Kinds of Providers*

QUALIFIER	PROVIDER
DN	Referring Provider: The physician who requests the service for the patient.
DK	Ordering Provider: A physician or, when appropriate, a non-physician who orders non-physician services for the patient. These services include diagnostic laboratory tests, clinical laboratory tests, pharmaceutical services, or durable medical equipment.
DQ	Supervising Provider: The physician monitoring the patient's care.

BLOCK 17A Leave blank.

BLOCK 17B This is where the National Provider Identifier (NPI) number of the referring, ordering, or supervising practitioner goes. As part of the enrollment process, all providers must apply for an NPI number. Authorized under the HIPAA Simplification Rule, the NPI is a unique identification number for all HIPAA-covered entities, including individuals, organizations, home health agencies, clinics, nursing homes, residential treatment homes, laboratories, ambulances, group practices, and health maintenance organizations (HMOs).

National Provider Identifier (NPI). Unique 10-digit code for providers required by HIPAA.

health maintenance organization (HMO). Plan that allows patients to only go to physicians, other health care professionals, or hospitals on a list of approved providers, except in an emergency.

BLOCK 18   Dates entered in either a six- or eight-digit format when a medical service rendered is a result of, or subsequent to, a related hospitalization.

EXAMPLE 2.5 *CMS-1500 Form Blocks 19-23*

19. ADDITIONAL CLAIM INFORMATION (Designated by NUCC)	20. OUTSIDE LAB? $ CHARGES
	☐ YES ☐ NO
21. DIAGNOSIS OR NATURE OF ILLNESS OR INJURY Relate A-L to service line below (24E) ICD Ind.	22. RESUBMISSION CODE ORIGINAL REF. NO.
A. B. C. D.	
E. F. G. H.	23. PRIOR AUTHORIZATION NUMBER
I. J. K. L.	
24 A DATE(S) OF SERVICE B C D. PROCEDURES, SERVICES, OR SUPPLIES E F G H I J Z	

Source: National Uniform Claim Committee

BLOCK 19   This block is used in numerous ways, based on the circumstances and payer type. Some common examples include:

- When modifier 99 (multiple modifiers) is used in block 24D, an explanation is given here in block 19 (e.g., 99 = 52 80 LT).

- When a claim needs to have a report or other documentation attached, enter "Additional Claim Information" in this block.

- Some payers require qualifiers in this block. Check with your private payer to see if this is required. NUCC provides a complete list on its website.

- Worker's Compensation requires additional information in this block. Each state has an official website for Worker's Compensation, with claim form instructions. NUCC also lists the qualifiers used.

- Medicare also has specific instructions for various situations and specialty claims. Complete instructions can be found at www.cms.gov.

BLOCK 20   Mark "yes" to the question asked if lab tests were done by an entity other than the one doing the billing. If multiple tests are involved, each should be filed under a separate claim.

BLOCK 21   Diagnosis codes go here.

BLOCK 22   Carrier-specific block; use for Medicaid claims.

BLOCK 23   The Quality Improvement Organization (QIO) prior authorization number goes here for those procedures that require it. Enter the Investigational Device Exemption (IDE) when an investigation device is used in an FDA-approved clinical trial.

Other information entered here includes the following.

- The NPI of a home health agency or hospice when either is billed

- The 10-digit Clinical Laboratory Improvement Act (CLIA) certification number for laboratory services billed by an entity performing CLIA-covered procedures

- The ZIP code of a loaded ambulance's point of pick-up

Important: Only one of these conditions can be listed per claim. If more than one applies, separate claims need to be submitted.

EXAMPLE 2.6 *CMS-1500 Form Blocks 24A-J*

24. A. DATE(S) OF SERVICE						B. PLACE OF SERVICE	C. EMG	D. PROCEDURES, SERVICES, OR SUPPLIES (Explain Unusual Circumstances)		E. DIAGNOSIS POINTER	F. $ CHARGES	G. DAYS OR UNITS	H. EPSDT Family Plan	I. ID. QUAL.	J. RENDERING PROVIDER ID. #
From MM	DD	YY	To MM	DD	YY			CPT/HCPCS	MODIFIER						
1														NPI	
2														NPI	
3														NPI	
4														NPI	
5														NPI	
6														NPI	

| 25. FEDERAL TAX I.D. NUMBER | SSN EIN | 26. PATIENT'S ACCOUNT NO. | 27. ACCEPT ASSIGNMENT? | 28. TOTAL CHARGE | 29. AMOUNT PAID | 30. Rsvd for NUCC Use |

PHYSICIAN OR SUPPLIER INFORMATION

Source: National Uniform Claim Committee

BLOCK 24A   Dates of service are listed here. Enter "From" and "To" dates in either a MMDDYY or MMDDCCYY format. When "From" and "To" dates are shown for a series of identical services, list them as a series of days in column G.

BLOCK 24B   This is where places of service codes go. These must be HIPAA-compliant. Codes are shown as two-digit numbers. For example, "01" should be used for a pharmacy, 02 is an unassigned number, 03 is for a school, and 04 is for a homeless shelter. CMS provides a complete list of blocks on its website, www.cms.gov.

BLOCK 24C   Carrier-specific block; used by Medicaid. Enter an "x" when billing for emergency services, or the claim may be reduced or denied.

BLOCK 24D   Enter procedures, services, and supplies. For this field, use CPT or HCPCS codes. These will be described in Chapter 5. This is also the place where modifiers go. Modifiers are additional information about types of services, such as surgical care or outpatient services. Modifiers are part of valid CPT or HCPCS codes.

BLOCK 24E   This field is for the diagnosis reference code (also known as the diagnosis pointer), as shown in Block 21. This field matches the date of service to the procedures performed under the primary diagnosis code. Enter only one reference number per line. Do not enter the diagnosis code here.

BLOCK 24F   Enter the provider's billed charges for each service.

BLOCK 24G   Enter the number of days or units. This field is mostly used for multiple visits, units of supplies, anesthesia minutes, or oxygen volume. If only one service is performed, the number "1" must be entered.

BLOCK 24H   Carrier-specific block. For Medicaid claims, refer to the Family Planning section of the Medicaid Providers Manual for detailed instructions.

BLOCK 24I   Enter the ID qualifier 1C in the shaded portion.

BLOCK 24J   Enter the rendering provider's NPI in the unshaded portion.

procedure code. ICD procedure codes (ICD-10-PCS), Current Procedural Terminology (CPT) codes, or the Healthcare Common Procedures Coding System (HCPCS) that represents the procedure or service.

modifier. Additional information about types of services, and part of valid CPT or HCPCS codes.

EXAMPLE 2.7 *CMS-1500 Form Blocks 25-33A*

25. FEDERAL TAX I.D. NUMBER	SSN EIN	26. PATIENT'S ACCOUNT NO.	27. ACCEPT ASSIGNMENT? (For govt. claims, see back)	28. TOTAL CHARGE	29. AMOUNT PAID	30. Rsvd for NUCC Use
	☐ ☐		☐ YES ☐ NO	$	$	
31. SIGNATURE OF PHYSICIAN OR SUPPLIER INCLUDING DEGREES OR CREDENTIALS (I certify that the statements on the reverse apply to this bill and are made a part thereof.) SIGNED DATE		32. SERVICE FACILITY LOCATION INFORMATION		33. BILLING PROVIDER INFO & PH # ( )		
		a. NPI	b.	a. NPI	b.	

Source: National Uniform Claim Committee

BLOCK 25 Enter the provider's or supplier's federal ID number or Social Security number and check the appropriate box.

BLOCK 26 Enter the patient's account number as assigned by the provider or supplier.

BLOCK 27 Check the appropriate box to indicate whether the provider or supplier accepts assignment of benefits. Be aware of which providers can only be paid on an assignment basis.

BLOCK 28 Enter total charges for all services.

BLOCK 29 For secondary claims only. Enter the total amount the patient's primary insurance paid.

BLOCK 30 Leave blank.

BLOCK 31 Enter the signature of the provider or the signature of an authorized representative.

BLOCK 32 Enter the name, address, and ZIP code of the facility where services were rendered.

BLOCK 32A Enter the NPI of the facility.

BLOCK 33 The provider's or supplier's billing name, address, ZIP code, and telephone number.

BLOCK 33A The NPI of the billing provider or group.

SUMMARY

This chapter has covered the following topics.

- A description of what information needs to go on a claim

- The difference between a clean and dirty claim

- Common mistakes made in filling out claims forms

- How to transmit claims

- The difference between primary and secondary insurance

- How to fill out the CMS-1500 form

In Chapter 3, you will learn what steps to take to avoid processing errors. The chapter includes a comprehensive list of front-end duties that can serve as a checklist of what you need to know and what needs to be done when preparing claims.

CHAPTER 2 DRILL QUESTIONS

Transmitting Claims

1. What is a claim?

2. Identify two items of information that need to be on a claim.

3. Which of the following describes a clean claim?

   a. All the data elements are completed.

   b. All the data elements are written on a white piece of paper.

   c. Almost all the data elements are right.

   d. All the necessary data elements are completed.

4. True or False: In 2012, the Administration Simplification Compliance Act (ASCA), part of HIPAA, mandated that health care claims be submitted electronically, with some exceptions.

CMS-1500 Form

5. The primary insurance plan does which of the following?

   a. Pays for everything

   b. Pays first

   c. Pays second

   d. Has the option of paying first or second

6. What is an NPI number? Where does it go on CMS-1500?

7. True or False: Misspelling a patient's name is a common processing error.

8. True or False: You are allowed to use both six- and eight-digits for the date on one claim.

9. Describe when Medicare is the secondary insurance for a patient.

10. By signing block 12 on the CMS-1500 form, a patient is doing which of the following?

    a. Authorizing the release of funds to a provider

    b. Authorizing the provider to perform a procedure

    c. Authorizing the release of medical information needed to process a claim

    d. Authorizing hospice care

CHAPTER 2 DRILL ANSWERS

1. A claim is a complete record of all the services provided to a patient.

2. Possible answers include the patient's name, health record number, account number, and demographic information, the subscriber number, group or plan number, and the provider's name.

3. **A.** *Incorrect* Some data elements should not be completed for a given claim, so this does not describe a clean claim.

   B. *Incorrect* A clean claim does not need to be written on a white piece of paper.

   C. *Incorrect* If any of the required information is inaccurate, then the claim would be considered dirty.

   D. *Correct* Clean claims are accurate and complete. They have all the information needed for processing.

4. True. One exception is if a provider uses a clearinghouse to submit claims. In this case, the draft sent to the clearinghouse may be completed on paper, and the correct form to use is CMS-1500.

5. **A.** *Incorrect* The primary insurance plan only pays up to the limit of its coverage.

   B. *Correct* The coordination of benefits rules determines which insurance plan is the primary plan, which is the one that pays first up to the limit of its coverage.

   C. *Incorrect* This describes the secondary insurance plan, which pays costs not covered by the primary plan.

   D. *Incorrect* The primary insurance plan does not have this option.

6. Authorized under the HIPAA Simplification Rule, the NPI is a unique identification number for all HIPAA-covered entities, including individuals, organizations, home health agencies, clinics, long-term care facilities, residential treatment centers, laboratories, ambulances, group practices, and health maintenance organizations (HMOs). NPI numbers go in blocks 17b, 19, 24J, 32A, and 33A.

7. True. Nicknames and hyphenated last names can complicate the task of getting the patient's name correct. Based on 2011 results, the average claims processing error rate was 19.3%.

8. False. You need to pick one style and use it throughout the claim.

9. Medicare is the secondary insurance for a patient when she has a group health insurance plan, is covered by workers' compensation, or is on disability.

10. **A.** *Incorrect* This is block 13 on the form.

    B. *Incorrect* This is not included on the CMS-1500 form.

    C. *Correct* Block 12 is an important field where the patient or an authorized person signs to authorize the release of medical information. The field must be dated and entered as a six- or eight-digit date. A signature on file or a computer-generated signature can also be used. The patient's signature authorizes release of information necessary to process the claim.

    D. *Incorrect* This is not included on the CMS-1500 form.

CHAPTER 3
Front-End Duties

OVERVIEW

Chapters 1 and 2 explained the importance of thorough, accurate health records. In Chapter 1, the emphasis was on complying with laws, many under the umbrella of the Health Insurance Portability and Accountability Act (HIPAA). In Chapter 2, the discussion centered on claims and claims processing. Claims are the way providers are reimbursed for their services. Accurate health records and health insurance information are the foundation of claims.

This chapter discusses steps that need to be taken to keep each patient's health insurance up-to-date and accurate. Tasks include verifying basic demographic and insurance information and ensuring that proper insurance verification, such as preauthorizations, precertifications, and predetermination are in place. To accomplish these tasks, it is important to know about the different health insurance plans available, as well as the difference between health maintenance organizations (HMOs) and preferred provider organizations (PPOs).

Once all the information has been gathered and verified as accurate, it is time to calculate the patient's balance due. That process involves verifying the patient's copayment, deductible, and coinsurance percentage. This information must be in place before a claim can be completed and sent to the appropriate insurance carrier.

COLLECTING PATIENT INFORMATION

Health organizations, such as hospitals, medical groups, and doctors' offices, have systems in place to collect patient information. In many organizations, the support staff or coding and billing staff are responsible for ensuring that the information in patient health insurance records is accurate and up-to-date.

In recent years, there has been a push to transfer all paper records into an electronic format. In most offices, information from forms filled out on paper is transferred to the electronic record. Many offices also provide patients with access to their health information through a secure portal. Using a login, patients can see their most recent health record. If patients catch any errors, they can inform the office staff.

By the end of this chapter, you should be able to answer the following questions.

1. Name three kinds of insurance information that needs to be collected from the patient.

2. Coordination of benefits involves which of the following?
   a. Double-checking each patient's insurance information
   b. Collecting demographic information
   c. Determining which insurance is primary and which is secondary
   d. Submitting a claim

3. True or False: The birthday rule is a way to mark how long a patient has had his insurance policy.

4. What is the difference between Medicare and Medicaid?

5. What is the advantage of employer-based self-insured health plans?

6. Which of the following accurately defines preauthorization?
   a. A doctor is given the go-ahead to see a patient.
   b. A physician suggests that a patient see a specialist.
   c. A health plan gives approval for an inpatient hospital stay or a surgical procedure.
   d. A hospital gives the doctor approval to perform a procedure.

7. Which of the following accurately describes a deductible?
   a. The cost of a health insurance premium
   b. A patient's share of the cost of health insurance
   c. The fee a patient pays for a doctor's visit
   d. The amount the patient must pay before the insurance company will start to provide benefits

8. True or False: A copay is the patient's share of the insurance premium.

9. Name one advantage and one disadvantage of a PPO.

10. What is the coinsurance percentage?

Collecting Basic Information

To collect basic information, such as a patient's demographic information, the first place to go is to the patient and family. When patients arrive at the hospital, a provider's office, or other facility, the following information is typically requested.

- Demographics
  - Name (first, middle initial, last)
  - Date of birth
  - Gender
  - Social Security number (last four digits)

This information will be compared to what is in the medical record or financial record. If the information does not match, flags can show up to indicate a possible problem. Then further verification can be requested, such as the patient's mother's maiden name.

What are two pieces of information that need to be collected from patients?

ANSWER: The patient's name (first name, middle initial, last name) and date of birth.

INSURANCE ELIGIBILITY

The support staff also needs to verify the patient's health insurance. As a first step, the staff member asks to see the patient's health insurance card to compare it to the information on file. The staff member may make a photocopy of the most recent card.

To verify benefits, the staff member calls the insurance company to double-check that the insurance information is valid. Before starting the conversation, it is essential to write down the name of the person who is providing this information.

Insurance information requested includes the following.

- Correct policy number and group number if applicable.
- Policy effective dates.
- Type of policy.
- Which benefit covers the primary treatment the patient is receiving.
- Policy limitations, such as the capitation (the fixed amount a provider receives), the policy's maximum benefit, and how much of the maximum the patient has already spent.
- Policy exclusions, such as specific products and services that are excluded from coverage.
- Deductible amounts, how much the patient has already satisfied, and the start date of the deductible period.

demographic information. Date of birth, sex, marital status, address, telephone number, relationship to subscriber, and circumstances of condition.

capitation. The fixed amount a provider receives.

- Coinsurance and copayments. *Note:* Deductibles, coinsurance, and copayments will be discussed later in this chapter.

- The address and phone of the insurance company to receive the claim.

- Whether prior authorization is required for any or all services. If so, case management (a review of the clinical services being performed) can be required as well.

- If the provider is out-of-network (not contracted with the health plan), deductibles and copays might be different. In some instances, no coverage will be available for out-of-network providers.

- Billing requirement for type of claim form and coding.

- Timely filing requirements for claim filing.

- Documentation requirements.

> *deductible.* The amount of money a patient must pay out of pocket before the insurance company will start to pay for covered benefits.

> *coinsurance.* The pre-established percentage of expenses paid by the insurance company after the deductible has been met.

> *copayment.* A fixed dollar amount that must be paid each time a patient visits a provider.

Other Patient Insurance Issues

In addition to verifying each patient's insurance information, there are a few other factors that affect billing. The first involves how many insurance plans a patient has. If she has more than one, it is necessary to determine which is the primary plan and which is the secondary plan. This process is called coordination of benefits. Going through this process ensures that there is no duplication in the payment of benefits. Typically, the primary insurance pays first. If the service was a covered benefit under the second plan, then it pays the balance. But third-party payers cannot collect more money than the provider charged for services.

> *coordination of benefits rules.* Determines which insurance plan is primary and which is secondary.

Birthday Rule

This informal procedure has been widely adopted by the insurance industry. It applies to dependent children whose parents have more than one insurance policy. Under the birthday rule, the health plan of the parent whose birthday comes first in the calendar year is designated as the primary plan. Note that it does not matter how old each parent is.

Some exceptions to the birthday rule are listed below.

1. If both parents have the same birthday, the health plan that has covered the parent the longest is considered the primary plan.

2. If the parents are separated or divorced, the health plan of the parent who has custody of the child is considered the primary plan. If one spouse has insurance under a group plan and the other spouse has an individual plan, the group plan is primary.

3. If one parent is employed and has a health insurance plan and the other parent has insurance through a former employer (such as through the Consolidated Omnibus Budget Reconciliation Act [COBRA]) and the children are listed as dependents on both plans, the plan of the active employee is the primary plan.

Third-Party Liability Insurance

If an accident has occurred, the third-party liability insurance should be filed as primary. These include the following.

- Automobile insurance policy
- Worker's compensation insurance
- Homeowner's insurance
- Malpractice insurance
- Business liability insurance

Medicare vs. Medicaid

For patients enrolled in both Medicare and Medicaid, Medicare always pays for services first. Medicaid is referred to as the payer of last resort.

Why is it important to verify insurance information?

ANSWER: Before submitting a claim, it is important to make sure that the insurance is valid and the services are a covered benefit.

What is the birthday rule?

ANSWER: The birthday rule applies to parents who both have health insurance and list their children as dependents. The health plan of the parent whose birthday comes first in the calendar year is considered primary and will be billed first for insurance claims.

GOVERNMENT AND COMMERCIAL INSURANCE

People have several options for health insurance. The government offers programs for specific population groups. Medicare is for people age 65 and those who are disabled. Medicaid is for low-income families and individuals.

The remaining population may obtain insurance through non-government carriers. Most people, however, get their insurance through commercial sources. They can purchase private insurance through an insurance company. Their health care is subsidized through premiums paid directly to the company.

Another option is to get health insurance through employers. These plans are self-insured by the employer and tend to be lower because additional fees are not built into the premiums. Employers budget a certain amount for employees' claims, which employers pay as they come in.

The next section describes these options in more detail.

---

third-party payer. Organization other than a patient who pays for services, such as insurance companies, Medicare, and Medicaid.

Government Insurance

Medicare

Medicare is health insurance provided to people age 65 or older, people younger than 65 who have certain disabilities, and people of all ages with end-stage kidney disease.

Medicare has the following four parts.

Medicare Part A provides hospitalization coverage, generally free of charge with a deductible, to individuals eligible for the Medicare benefit. Health care services covered include inpatient hospital care, skilled nursing facility care, home health care, hospice care, and inpatient care in a religious, nonmedical health care institution. Coverage for inpatient hospital stays and skilled nursing facility care are measured in benefit periods. A benefit period begins when the patient is admitted to a hospital or skilled nursing facility and ends when the patient has not received care for 60 consecutive days. There are limitations on how much Medicare Part A pays for each kind of service.

Under ***Medicare Part B***, people can purchase voluntary supplemental medical insurance (SMI) to help pay for physicians' and other medical professionals' services, medical services, and medical-surgical supplies not covered by Medicare Part A with a calendar deductible and 20% coinsurance of Medicare's allowable charge for most services.

Other services covered include the following.

- Care provided at an emergency department or outpatient clinic, such as same-day surgery

- Home health care not covered under Part A

- Laboratory tests, x-rays, and other diagnostic radiology services

- Ambulatory surgery center services at Medicare-approved facilities

- Most physical, speech, and occupational therapy services

- Radiation therapy, kidney dialysis, and transplants

- Heart and liver transplants

- Inpatient hospitalizations when Part A benefits have been exhausted

Services not covered by Part A or Part B include the following.

- Long-term nursing care

- Cosmetic surgery

- Dentures and dental care

- Acupuncture

- Hearing aids and exams for fitting hearing aids

Medicare Part A. Provides hospitalization insurance to eligible individuals.

Medicare Part B. Voluntary supplemental medical insurance to help pay for physicians' and other medical professionals' services, medical services, and medical-surgical supplies not covered by Medicare Part A.

Medicare Advantage (MA) plans offer a combined package of the benefits under both Parts A and B. In some instances, they may offer extra coverage for services such as vision, hearing, dental, or health and wellness programs. Many also include prescription drug coverage. Organizations offering MA plans must meet specific requirements from the Centers for Medicare and Medicaid Services (CMS).

The following options are available through Medicare Advantage.

- Health maintenance organizations (HMOs) allow patients to only go to physicians, other health care professionals, or hospitals on the plan's list of approved providers, except in an emergency.

- Preferred provider organizations (PPOs) allow patients to use doctors, specialists, and hospitals in the plan's network. Going to doctors and hospitals not on the list usually means that patients will have to pay extra.

- Private fee-for-service plans allow patients to go to any physician, other health care professional, or hospital as long as the providers agree to treat those patients. The plan determines how much it will pay providers and how much patients must pay for care.

- Medicare specialty plans provide focused, specialized health care for specific groups of people, such as those who have both Medicare and Medicaid, live in a nursing home, or have chronic medical conditions.

Medicare Part D pays for medications. The drug benefit is run by private insurance companies and other vendors approved by Medicare. There are many plans to choose from, and they can vary in cost and drugs covered. Beneficiaries can choose the plan that best meets their needs.

Out-of-pocket expenses are applied to individuals who elect the traditional Medicare Parts A, B, and D. Patients are responsible for charges not covered by Medicare, as well as for various cost-sharing requirements of Parts A and B. These expenses can be paid by the Medicare beneficiary, an employer-sponsored health, or Medigap, a private health insurance that pays for most of the charges not covered by Parts A and B. If a beneficiary is eligible for Medicaid, it could pay for some of the outstanding expenses not covered by Medicare.

Medicare Advantage (MA). Combined package of benefits under Medicare Parts A and B that may offer extra coverage for services such as vision, hearing, dental, health and wellness, or prescription drug coverage.

Medicare Part D. A plan run by private insurance companies and other vendors approved by Medicare.

Medigap. A private health insurance that pays for most of the charges not covered by Parts A and B.

Medicaid

This government-based health insurance option is funded through a partnership between state governments and the federal Medicaid program. The program pays for medical assistance for individuals with low incomes and limited financial resources.

To participate in Medicaid, states must meet guidelines established by federal laws, regulations, and policies. If the states meet those requirements, they qualify for federal matching grants. Each state has its own agency that determines Medicaid eligibility for residents. Medicaid policies vary from state to state, so a person eligible in one state might not be eligible in another. However, the federal government has established that the following are considered categorically needy eligible groups.

- Those who meet the requirements for Temporary Assistance for Needy Families (TANF)

- Children younger than 6 years whose family income is 133% or less of the federal poverty level

- Pregnant women whose family income is below 133% of the federal poverty level

- Supplemental Security Income recipients (in most states)

- Recipients of adoption or foster care assistance

- Individuals who lose their cash assistance due to earnings from work or increased Social Security benefits

- Infants born to Medicaid-eligible women

- Certain low-income Medicare recipients

Services covered under Medicaid. To receive federal matching funds, a state must provide the following services.

- Inpatient hospital care

- Outpatient hospital care

- Emergency care

- Prenatal care

- Vaccines for children

- Physicians' services

- Skilled nursing facilities services for persons 2 years of age or older

- Family planning services and supplies

- Rural health clinic services

- Home health care for persons eligible for skilled nursing services;

- Laboratory and x-ray services

- Pediatric and family nurse practitioner services

- Nurse-midwife services

- Federally qualified health center services and ambulatory services performed at a federally qualified health center that would be available in other settings

- Early and periodic screening, diagnosis, and therapeutic (EPSDT) services for patients under age 21

States may also receive federal matching funds to provide some of the following optional services.

- Diagnostic services

- Clinic services

- Prescription drugs and prosthetic devices

- Transportation services

- Rehabilitation and physical therapy services

- Home care and community-based care services for chronic impairments

State Children's Health Insurance Program (SCHIP)

This program is jointly funded by the federal government and the states. States must meet the following three eligibility criteria.

1. Recipients must come from low-income families.

2. Recipients must be otherwise ineligible for Medicaid.

3. Recipients must be uninsured.

States must offer the following services.

- Inpatient hospital care

- Outpatient hospital care

- Physicians' surgical and medical services

- Laboratory and x-ray services

- Well baby/child care, including age-appropriate immunizations

Commercial Insurance

This refers to two kinds of insurance: private and employer-based self-insurance. Private insurance is paid for by the individual, while employer-based self-insurance is tied to an individual's place of employment. Both kinds of commercial insurance are explained in the following sections.

Private Health Insurance Plans

These plans are paid for through premiums, which are a pre-established amount set by the insurance company and paid regularly, usually on a monthly basis. The premiums of all the plan's participants go into a special fund, which is used to pay for claims. Before paying a claim, the company reviews it carefully to make sure the service is covered by the plan. Reviewers also check the diagnosis codes to make sure the services were medically necessary. Payment is made to either the provider or the policyholder.

Up-front information provided to the policyholder before signing on to a plan includes the following.

- What medical services will be covered

- When the company will pay for those medical services

- How much and for how long the company will pay for the covered services

- Which process is to be followed to ensure that covered medical expenses are paid

Employer-Based Self-Insurance Plans

Companies save money by self-insuring their employee health plans rather than purchasing coverage from private insurance companies. Self-insurance costs are lower because additional fees built into premiums by private insurers are eliminated.

Employer-based self-insurance plans vary in design and what services are covered. Many have a cost-sharing feature, where expenses are shared with employees and are taken out of their paychecks each pay period. But due to economies of scale, costs of employer-based health insurance plans tend to be lower than those purchased by individuals.

Plans are usually funded through administrative services only (ASO) contracts between employers and private insurers. Under these contracts, employers fund the plans themselves, and the private insurers administer the plans for the employers.

Blue Cross and Blue Shield Plans

These plans were the first prepaid plans in the U.S. Originally, Blue Cross covered hospital care and Blue Shield covered physicians' services. They merged to form the Blue Cross and Blue Shield Association (BC/BS) in 1982.

BC/BS, also called the Blues, includes more than 60 independent, locally operated companies with plans in 50 states, the District of Columbia, and Puerto Rico. The Blues offer health insurance to individuals, small businesses, seniors, and large employer groups. The federal government also has a large program called the BC/BS Federal Employee Program.

What are the three major kinds of government insurance plans?

ANSWER: Medicare, Medicaid, and State Children's Health Insurance Program (SCHIP).

What is the difference between private health insurance and employer self-insured plans?

ANSWER: Private health insurance is paid by individuals in the form of premiums to the insurance company. Employer self-insured plans are purchased in mass by the employer and can be more cost-effective. Additional costs added to premiums are largely eliminated, and employers fund the health insurance plans. Often, employers enter into agreements with private insurers to manage the plans.

PATIENT AUTHORIZATION AND REFERRAL FORMS

Much of the up-front paperwork is done to determine whether a specific medical or surgical procedure is needed and to receive the necessary approvals from the health insurance plan. Different plans have different procedures in place and may use different terms to describe similar processes. For these reasons, understanding what steps need to be taken can be confusing.

Therefore, patient authorizations and referrals are explained in terms of types of health plans. The two major categories are HMOs and PPOs. Both are considered managed care organizations, which were developed to manage the quality of health care and control costs. For example, utilization review, a process used to determine the medical necessity of a particular procedure or service, was designed to ensure that the procedure or service is appropriate and is being provided in the most cost-effective way. Over time, other cost controls were incorporated in health plans in specific ways.

HMOs

There are four different kinds of HMOs: the staff model, group practice model, network model, and independent practice association (IPA). While each is unique, they share the following characteristics.

- They are organized systems of health care delivery for a specific geographic area.

- They have an established set of basic and supplemental health maintenance and treatment services.

- They have members who enroll voluntarily.

- They offer predetermined, fixed, and periodic prepayments for enrollees.

Staff Model

The HMO staff model provides hospitalization and physician services through its own staff. Typically, this type of HMO owns its facility. The physicians are employees of the HMO who are either paid a salary or on a predetermined fixed amount per member per month. The latter approach is called capitation.

Enrollees have the least amount of control of the providers under this plan compared to any other. Referrals, or written recommendations to specialists, are confined to those within the HMO staff. In addition, any referrals are strictly controlled by the primary care physicians (PCPs), which is referred to as the gatekeeper model. Services received outside this kind of HMO must be paid out of pocket by the patient.

Group Practice Model

The group practice model is different from the staff model in that the HMO contracts with an outside medical group for services. The health care professionals are paid on a capitation basis.

Network Model

The network model is similar to the group model, with one key exception: the HMO contracts with two or more independent practices. This provides greater choice to enrollees in the HMO. With both group practice and network HMOs, referral from the provider is needed for specialists (gatekeeper model).

IPA Model

In the IPA model, the HMO contracts with the IPA, which in turn contracts with individual health providers. The HMO reimburses the IPA on a capitated basis, and the IPA in turn may reimburse the physicians on a capitated or fee-for-service basis. The participating physicians see patients who are part of the HMO and those who are not.

---

referral. Written recommendation to a specialist.

PPOs

PPOs contract with employers and insurers to provide health care services to a group of members. PPOs are more flexible and have a broader network from which members can choose providers. But because of this flexibility, they also have mechanisms in place to control costs.

In some PPOs, the PCP serves as the gatekeeper for services. The PCP determines whether the referral to specialists, other health care sites for diagnostic or therapeutic procedures, hospitals, or other health care facilities are warranted. Gatekeepers determine the appropriateness of the health care service, level of health care professional called for, and setting for care.

For some health care services, such as surgery or a hospital stay, prior approval (preauthorization) is required. Preauthorization is when the health plan is notified that a hospital stay is coming up, giving the plan the opportunity to determine if the hospital stay is medically necessary and how many days the patient most likely will need to stay. Most health insurance cards list a phone number for preauthorization services and when preauthorization is required. A preauthorization number is provided when the health care services are approved.

Some plans call a similar process precertification. This, too, is done before a procedure or surgery is performed. This review looks at whether the procedure could be performed safely but less expensively in an outpatient setting. If the insurance plan thinks the service is unwarranted, it can deny coverage. If approved, the plan will provide a precertification number.

precertification. A review that looks at whether the procedure could be performed safely but less expensively in an outpatient setting.

Another form of approval is predetermination. This refers to a written request for a verification of benefits. The insurance plan sends back, in writing, an explanation of the health benefits. Patients can request a predetermination of benefits before undergoing a medical procedure, but usually this is not necessary.

predetermination. A written request for a verification of benefits.

Who is usually the gatekeeper, and what is that individual's role?

ANSWER: The gatekeeper is usually the primary care physician. The gatekeeper determines if referrals to specialists, services, or facilities are needed and then selects the provider the patient should go to.

What is preauthorization?

ANSWER: Preauthorization is approval from the health plan for an inpatient hospital stay or surgery. Before giving approval, the health plan will assess whether the procedure is medically necessary and how long the hospital stay should be.

DETERMINING BALANCE DUE

To figure out the balance owed from patients, it is necessary to understand the "fine print" of their insurance plans. Most plans have cost-sharing provisions, which help determine how much the insurance will pay and how much the patients owe. Cost-sharing provisions usually involve deductibles, copayments, and the coinsurance percentage.

Deductibles

Deductibles refer to the amount of money patients must pay out of pocket before the insurance company will start to pay for covered benefits. Deductibles vary considerably from plan to plan. Some may be $500 for an individual to as much as $1,000. For a family, the range can vary from $1,000 to $2,000. The deductible must be met for each calendar year. Any expenses not covered will be applied to the deductible.

Copayments

Copayments are a fixed dollar amount, often called a flat fee, which must be paid each time a patient visits a provider. Copayments vary from provider to provider. A visit to an outpatient clinic might have a $15 copay, while the copay for outpatient surgery can be $50.

Prescriptions also have variable copayments. Insurance companies usually have a list of prescription drugs covered, called a formulary. The least expensive drugs in the formulary are generics, or those not covered by a patent. This level is referred to as Tier 1. The next level, Tier 2, is a nongeneric prescription drug with a preferred brand name. Tier 3 is a prescription drug with a nonpreferred brand name, and Tier 4 is not on the formulary. In general, the cheapest option, with the lowest copayment, is the generic drug.

formulary. A list of prescription drugs covered by an insurance plan.

Tier 1. Providers and facilities in a PPO's network.

Tier 2. Providers and facilities within a broader, contracted network of the insurance company.

Tier 3. Providers and facilities out of the network.

Tier 4. Providers and facilities not on the formulary.

preferred provider. Tier 2 provider.

Medical services may also be placed in a tier system by the insurance company. Tier 1 providers and facilities are in the PPO's network and are the least expensive, with the patient paying the lowest premium and the copay. Under this option, the PCP coordinates and authorizes all of the patient's health care services.

Tier 2 refers to providers and facilities within a broader, contracted network of the insurance company. These providers are called preferred providers. Under this option, no individual physician coordinates the member's health care services. Usually, the member pays a mid-range premium, deductible, and coinsurance.

Tier 3 refers to providers and facilities out of the network. This is the most expensive option, but provides members with the freedom to choose any health care professional they want. These members have the highest deductibles, coinsurance, and copayments.

Coinsurance

Coinsurance, sometimes referred to as the rate of payment, is the pre-established percentage of expenses paid by the insurance company after the deductible has been met. Many plans have a 80/20 formula in place, meaning that the insurance company pays 80% of the costs and the member pays 20%. For example, if a cost of a medical service is $500, the insurance company pays $400 and the member pays $100.

Many plans have a maximum in place. That means that after the members have reached a predetermined amount, the insurance company will pay 100% of the cost of the medical service. For example, a health plan could establish $5,000 as its maximum amount.

What's the difference between a copayment and coinsurance?

ANSWER: A copayment is a flat fee that a patient pays for visiting a provider or purchasing prescription drugs. The copayment varies from provider to provider. Coinsurance is a percentage of the covered benefits paid by both the insurance company and the patient. Many insurance companies pay 80% of the covered benefits, with the patient paying the remaining 20%.

SUMMARY

This chapter has covered the following points.

- What information about the patient and insurance plan needs to be collected up front

- Types of government-based insurance options

- Types of private insurance

- The difference between HMOs and PPOs

- The kinds of forms that may be requested, including preauthorization, precertification, and predetermination

- Cost-control mechanisms in place, including deductibles, copayments, and the coinsurance percentage

The next chapter explains how to interpret information received from the insurance company after a claim is processed. This includes understanding how to interpret the remittance advice received from the insurance company to determine the financial responsibility of each party, as well as how to interpret denial codes, which offer some explanation about why a claim was denied. These steps help ensure that both the insurance companies and patients are paying their fair share.

CHAPTER 3 DRILL QUESTIONS

Collecting Patient Information

1. Name three kinds of insurance information that needs to be collected from the patient.

Insurance Eligibility

2. Coordination of benefits involves which of the following?

   a. Double-checking each patient's insurance information

   b. Collecting demographic information

   c. Determining which insurance is primary and which is secondary

   d. Submitting a claim

3. True or False: The birthday rule is a way to mark how long a patient has had his insurance policy.

Government and Commercial Insurance

4. What is the difference between Medicare and Medicaid?

5. What is the advantage of employer-based self-insured health plans?

Patient Authorization and Referral Forms

6. Which of the following accurately defines preauthorization?

   a. A doctor is given the go-ahead to see a patient.

   b. A physician suggests that a patient see a specialist.

   c. A health plan gives approval for an inpatient hospital stay or a surgical procedure.

   d. A hospital gives the doctor approval to perform a procedure.

Determining Balance Due

7. Which of the following accurately describes a deductible?

   a. The cost of a health insurance premium

   b. A patient's share of the cost of health insurance

   c. The fee a patient pays for a doctor's visit

   d. The amount the patient must pay before the insurance company will start to provide benefits

8. True or False: A copay is the patient's share of the insurance premium.

9. Name one advantage and one disadvantage of a PPO.

10. What is the coinsurance percentage?

CHAPTER 3 DRILL ANSWERS

1. Among the correct responses are the correct policy number and group number, if applicable; policy effective dates; and type of policy.

2. **A.** *Incorrect* This is a good practice, but it does not apply to coordination of benefits.
    B. *Incorrect* Collecting demographic information is an important part of capturing the appropriate health insurance information, but it is not related to coordination of benefits.
    C. *Correct* The coordination of benefits process, which determines primary and secondary insurance, ensures that there is no duplication in the payment of benefits. The primary insurance pays first, up to its coverage limits, and the secondary insurance pays second.
    D. *Incorrect* Coordination of benefits should be determined prior to submitting a claim.

3. False. The birthday rule is a way to determine primary insurance if both parents have insurance and list their children as dependents. The insurance of the parent whose birthday is first in the calendar year is considered the primary insurance.

4. Medicare is a government-based insurance plan that covers people older than 65, those younger than 65 with disabilities, and those with end-stage kidney disease. Medicaid covers low-income families and individuals.

5. Due to economies of scale, employer-based self-insured health plans are more reasonably priced than private insurance.

6. **A.** *Incorrect* Preauthorization does not refer to authorization for a doctor to see a patient.
    B. *Incorrect* This describes a referral.
    C. *Correct* For some health care services, such as surgery or a hospital stay, prior approval is required. Preauthorization is when the health plan is notified that a hospital stay is coming up, giving the plan the opportunity to determine if the hospital stay is medically necessary and how many days the patient most likely will need to stay.
    D. *Incorrect* Preauthorization does not refer to authorization given by a hospital to a doctor.

7. **A.** *Incorrect* A health insurance premium is not the same as a deductible.
    B. *Incorrect* A deductible makes up only part of the patient's share of the cost of health insurance.
    C. *Incorrect* This refers to a copayment.
    D. *Correct* This correctly describes deductibles, which vary considerably from plan to plan. The deductible must be met for each calendar year. Any expenses not covered will be applied to the deductible.

8. False. Insurance premium is a weekly, monthly, or annual cost for the plan or insurance coverage. Copayment is the out-of-pocket cost.

9. PPOs generally provide greater choice in the health care professionals patients can choose to see. Patients do not need a referral from the provider to see a specialist. A disadvantage is that cost-control measures, such as coinsurance and copayments, are usually in place.

10. The coinsurance percentage is the amount the provider is allowed for the service and the amount he was paid. The patient has coinsurance responsibility to what provider was allowed. A common percentage split is 80% for the insurance carrier and 20% for the patient.

CHAPTER 4
Payment Adjudication

OVERVIEW

Chapters 2 and 3 focused on how to submit a claim and what tasks have to be completed to ensure that the submission process goes smoothly. This chapter covers what happens after the claim is submitted. Many steps take place at this point. While the third-party payer, or health insurer, is reviewing the claim, the accounts receivable department keeps track of what third-party payers the provider is waiting to hear from and what patients are due to make a payment.

During this time, the patient receives an explanation of benefits (EOB). The EOB describes the services rendered, payment covered, and benefit limits and denials. Medicare patients receive a similar document called the Medicare Summary Notice (MSN). Both documents prepare the patient for what bills to expect.

After the third-party payer has processed the claim, a remittance advice (RA) is sent back to the provider. Payments may accompany the RA. The RA also identifies claims that have been rejected or denied. Next, the health care facility determines the amount the patient owes. If the claim has been rejected or denied, the facility will have to address that as well. Once all payments have been received and issues resolved, the payment adjudication process is complete. This process is also called the revenue cycle. This chapter will go over each of these steps in more detail.

By the end of this chapter, you should be able to answer the following questions.

1. What is the role of the accounts receivable department?

2. What are two kinds of information the CDM stores?

3. An aging report refers to which of the following?
   a. The length of time the report has been in the CDM
   b. The ages of all patients in a provider's practice
   c. The claims that are outstanding
   d. The amount of money the provider's office has received in the last 6 months

4. True or False: An RA is sent to policyholders.

5. The allowable charge is which of the following?
   a. Amount the provider charges for a service
   b. Amount the patient agrees to pay
   c. Amount the health insurance company will pay providers
   d. Amount set by hospitals

6. Which of the following is NOT a charge the patient is expected to pay?
   a. Coinsurance
   b. Deductible
   c. Difference between a provider's charges and what the insurance company will pay
   d. Copayment

7. The term reconciliation means which of the following?
   a. Resolving difference with the insurance company
   b. Working with Medicare on a problem
   c. Getting more information about a patient from a physician
   d. Determining how much the provider has been reimbursed and how much patients owe

8. What are the four types of nonmedical codes used by Medicare to explain claims?

9. Who benefits from the new appeals process, and why?

10. When can a patient request an external independent review?

---

accounts receivable department. Department that keeps track of what third-party payers the provider is waiting to hear from and what patients are due to make a payment.

---

explanation of benefits (EOB). Describes the services rendered, payment covered, and benefit limits and denials.

ANALYZING AGING REPORTS

The accounts receivable department manages the billing process for the provider. This department tracks which patients have received services but not paid. This is usually because the provider is waiting to see the reimbursement amount received from the third-party payer.

The accounts receivable department also manages the charge description master (CDM). The CDM has all the information about health care services that patients have received and financial transactions that have taken place. The primary purpose of the CDM is to make sure that the provider accurately charges the patient for routine services and supplies.

Information in the CDM includes the following.

- Description of service can be an evaluation and management visit, observation, or emergency room visit.

- CPT/HCPCS code must correspond to the description of the service. (*Note:* Codes will be explained in Chapter 5.)

- Revenue code (also called the UB-04 code) is a three-digit code that describes a classification of a product or service provided to the patient. Revenue codes are required for Medicare patients.

- Charge amount is the amount the facility charges for the procedure or service. This amount is not necessarily what the facility will receive from the third-party payer.

- Charge or service code is an internally assigned number unique to each facility. It identifies each procedure listed on the charge. This code can be useful for revenue tracking.

- General ledger key is a two- or three-digit number that makes sure that a line item is assigned to the general ledger in the hospital's accounting system.

- Activity/status date indicates the most recent activity of an item.

It is important to keep the CDM accurate and up-to-date. Information in the CDM is often used as a source for the claim, so an inaccurate CDM could mean an inaccurate claim. Table 4.1 shows the kinds of problems that can occur when the CDM is not maintained.

TABLE 4.1 *Issues that are Tracked on the CDM*

ISSUE	POSSIBLE OUTCOME	POSSIBLE RISK
Undercharging for services	Underpayment	Lost revenue
Overcharging for services	Overpayment	Compliance
Incorrect HCPCS or diagnosis code	Claims rejection or denial	Lost revenue
Incorrect revenue code	Claims rejection or denial	Lost revenue

---

aging report. Measures the outstanding balances in each account.

---

charge description master (CDM). Information about health care services that patients have received and financial transactions that have taken place.

Managing Aging Reports

Another function of the accounts receivable department is managing aging reports, also known as age trial balance (ATB). In accounting, this term has a specific meaning that refers to the status of an invoice. The provider might be waiting for payments from the third-party payer, patient, or both.

The accounts receivable department uses a formula to calculate the number of days the claim is still open, or unresolved.

$$\frac{\text{Ending accounts receivable balance}}{\text{Average revenue per day}}$$

Aging reports are often maintained in 30-day increments. For example, a report of "0-30 days" means that invoices have gone past the due date by 0 to 30 days. A report of "31-60 days" means that invoices are past due by 31 to 60 days. Facilities monitor multiple accounts and the amount due in each one.

Assessing the Status of Accounts

Aging reports are useful because they help the office staff see which accounts have not been paid. By checking the EOB or RA, it is possible to tell why an account has an outstanding balance. Reasons for lack of payment include the following.

- The third-party payer has not processed the claim. The delay might be backed up on the insurance side, or the claim was not filled out correctly and could not be processed. If a claim has to be reviewed manually, that will also delay action on the claim.

- A patient has not paid his or her balance, and has not notified the office to say why.

- A claim is held up in the office because the provider has neglected to give the billing staff necessary information.

The office staff may set priorities about which accounts to address first. They may decide to prioritize accounts with high dollar amounts or those that are older when it's time to collect payments. This is because, in general, the older the account or the longer it remains unpaid, the less likely the facility will receive reimbursement from the third-party payer.

The office's priorities also may determine which of the above groups the staff is directed to contact first. It could be the third-party payer, patient, or a provider in the office. Appropriate follow-up includes the following.

- Contact the third-party payer(s) involved and find out why the claim has been delayed. If the third-party payer alerts the staff person to a problem, then the office will need to fix it. The problem might be a coding mistake or a problem with the patient's registration information. In many instances, it is possible to correct the mistake online and re-submit the claim.

- Call the patient to find out why payment has been delayed. If the patient is experiencing financial difficulties, it might be possible to work out a payment plan. If the patient is able but unwilling to pay, then medical offices may hire a collection agency to try to collect the outstanding balance. Although there is no fixed timeframe for bringing in a collection agency, most wait 90 to 120 days from the time the bill was issued before taking this step.

- Work with the health care professional in your office to get all the information needed for a claim. Query forms are available to help the billing staff communicate with physicians.

The following information should be included on the query form.

- Patient's name

- Service date

- Health record number

- Account number

- Date query initiated

- Name and contact information of the individual initiating the query

- Statement of the issue in the form of a question with specific information from the chart referenced

  ○ For example, a staff member might need to know what type of anemia a patient had in order to verify that the prescribed blood transfusion that was warranted.

After resolving these issues, complete the claim and submit it as soon as it is ready.

What is an aging report?

ANSWER: An aging report identifies the outstanding balances in each account. Aging reports are usually organized in 30-day increments. For example, a report of 0-30 days means that the invoice is past due by 0 to 30 days.

INTERPRETING REMITTANCE ADVICE

Remittance advice (RA) is the report sent from the third-party payer to the provider. A similar document, the explanation of benefits (EOB), is sent to the policyholder. Medicare Summary Notices (MSNs) are sent to Medicare patients. MSNs outline the amounts billed by the provider and what the patient must pay the provider, usually in the form of deductibles and copayments.

These documents are usually sent out at the same time. They explain how the third-party payer determined the payment the provider will receive and the balance the policyholder must pay.

account number. Number that identifies specific episode of care, date of service, or patient.

health record number. Number the provider uses to identify an individual patient's record.

Medicare Summary Notice (MSN). Document that outlines the amounts billed by the provider and what the patient must pay the provider.

Components of an RA

The following basic information is on a typical RA. Much of this information is also on an EOB, which the policyholder receives.

- Name of the health care insurance company

- Date of the report

- Name of the subscriber and her identification number, referred to as the certificate number or member number

- Subscriber's group number

- Name and address of provider, such as a medical office or a durable medical equipment vendor

FIGURE 4.1 *Remittance Advice Report Example*

Insurance
E X A M P L E

P. O. Box 99999
Anywhere, MO 12345
Customer Service 1.800.555.1234

Medicare Management Information System
Remittance Advice

Anytown Medical Group
123 Main Street
Small Town, KS 54321

Date	11/07/20XX
Remittance	1234567
Remit Seq	456
Page	1

Provider ID   MC44NP
NPI ID   1234567890
Subscriber   Carptenter, Molly A
Certificate ID 0789123456

Certificate ID	Code	Description	Billed Amt	Allowed	Due to Member	Status
0789123456	99171	Office visit	$40.00	$32.00	$8.00	
	87081	Culture, presumptive	$100.00	$80.00	$20.00	
Total			$140.00	$112.00	$28.00	UNPAID

RJH
ASSESSMENT TECHNOLOGIES INSTITUTE

- Health care services received and the date or dates

This information pertains to payment issues.

- Actual charge, also called the billed amount, refers to the amount the provider charges for the health care service. This amount might not be the same as the allowable charge. The actual charge may be subject to discounts.

- Allowable charge, also called allowable fee, maximum fee, maximum allowable, usual-reasonable-customary, UCR charge, or prevailing rate, is the amount the insurer will actually pay. Allowable charges include discounted fees, which the insurer negotiated with providers. Under such arrangements, providers agree to accept the allowable charge as the full payment. Each insurer has its own schedule of allowed charges. These charges are subject to deductibles, copayments, and coinsurance.

- Write-offs are the difference between the provider's actual charge and the allowable charge. Write-offs refer to the contracted discount rates. They are called write-offs because the provider has agreed to accept the allowable charge as the full payment minus any deductibles, copayments, and coinsurance. The provider "writes off" the excess amount.

- Cost sharing, such as deductibles, copayments, and coinsurance, are collected by the providers from the policyholders. This amount represents the balance the policyholder must pay to the provider.

- Rejections and denials need coding explaining the reasons. Insurance company denials will be explained later in this chapter.

subscriber. Purchaser of the insurance or the member of group for which an employer or association as purchased insurance.

subscriber number. Unique code used to identify a subscriber's policy.

cost sharing. The balance the policyholder must pay to the provider.

Other information on the RA includes the following.

- If claims were submitted in groups, often referred to as batches, the RA may include names of multiple patients and their account numbers. Sometimes the birthdates of patients are included as well.

- Prior approval number, either an authorization or a pre-certification number.

- Provider/practitioner number, in addition to the name and address.

- Tax identification number.

- Check number and amount.

- Payment due.

- Service code and modifiers, which will be explained in Chapter 5. This information also may be on the patient's EOB.

- Claim status: paid, denied or rejected, reversed (corrected), or suspended.

- Rejections, reversals, denials, disallowed charges, allowances, reason codes, and other details for multiple patients.

The RA, EOB, and MSN contain information needed to post payments to the appropriate parties. The provider's office takes care of this step, using these documents as a guide. The procedure for posting payments is described later in this chapter.

RAs for Medicare Participants

As providers enter arrangements with insurance companies stating they agree to the allowable charge, Medicare participants enter into similar arrangements. In this context, participating physicians accept assignment. This means that the health care professional accepts as payment in full Medicare's allowable charge.

batch. A group of submitted claims.

balance billing. Billing patients for charges in excess of the Medicare fee schedule.

Notice of Exclusions from Medicare Benefits. Notification by the physician to a patient that a service will not be paid.

Advance Beneficiary Notice of Noncoverage. Form provided if a provider believes that a service may be declined because Medicare might consider it unnecessary.

Health care professionals are prohibited from balance billing. This means that they can't bill patients for charges in excess of the Medicare fee schedule. However, providers are allowed to bill for services not covered by Medicare. Physicians must notify the patient that the service will not be paid by giving the patient a Notice of Exclusions from Medicare Benefits. If a provider believes that a service may be declined because Medicare might consider it unnecessary, the patient must be notified by sending out an Advance Beneficiary Notice of Noncoverage. This form is used mostly in home health settings and skilled nursing facilities.

What is the difference between an RA and an EOB?

ANSWER: The RA often includes more information than the EOB, including a breakdown of the allowable charge vs. the actual charge, write-offs, and information from multiple patients. The EOB is an explanation of the benefits applied for one policyholder. Both the RA and EOB contain information about the patient's responsibility for payment along with denied services and reimbursed services. RAs are primarily sent to providers and EOBs are primarily sent to the policyholder. However, there are times when these two terms are used interchangeably since the information on both documents is similar.

POSTING PAYMENTS

Posting payments, also called reconciliation and collections, is the final step in the revenue cycle. This is when the health care office or facility receives its reimbursement from the third-party payers and determines which accounts can be closed. It is also when the provider uses the RA, EOB, and MSN to identify the amount owed by the patient.

Accounts can also be reconciled through a write-off or an adjustment to a patient's account. This information is then entered into the billing software system. This record is a tool to track payments owed and claims rejections.

After the information is entered into the billing software, the billing department can send a bill to the patient for the amount owed. These payments can be the result of outstanding deductibles and copayments.

Once an account has been settled, the revenue cycle is considered complete. Figure. 4.2 illustrates the key parts of the revenue cycle.

FIGURE 4.2 *Revenue Cycle*

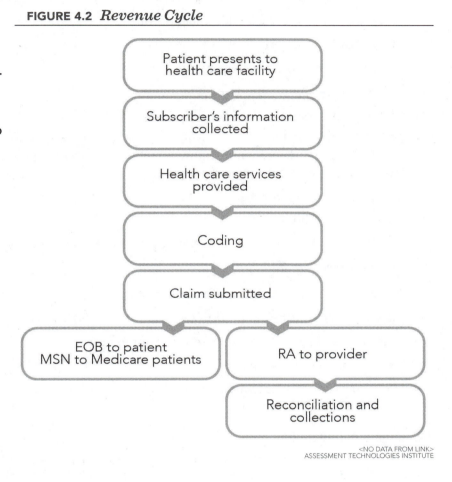

Patient presents to health care facility

Subscriber's information collected

Health care services provided

Coding

Claim submitted

EOB to patient
MSN to Medicare patients

RA to provider

Reconciliation and collections

<NO DATA FROM LINK>
ASSESSMENT TECHNOLOGIES INSTITUTE

What does the term reconciliation mean?

ANSWER: Reconciliation refers to the process the billing office goes through to determine what payments have come in from the third-party payer and what the patient owes the provider. The billing office uses the RA, EOB, and MSN to make these determinations.

write-off. The difference between the provider's actual charge and the allowable charge.

DETERMINING REASONS FOR INSURANCE COMPANY DENIAL

There are many possible reasons for a denial of a claim. Errors can occur at any point in the revenue cycle. The following are some common reasons.

- Differences in a patient's name or its spelling, such as a nickname or a hyphenated last name

- Missing or invalid patient identification number

- Missing or invalid patient information, such as sex, date of birth, or Social Security number

- Missing or invalid subscriber (member) name

- Missing or invalid certificate or group number

- Lack of authorization or referral number

- Failure to check the box for assignment of benefits (contract in which the provider directly bills the payer and accepts the allowable charge, or the amount the insurer will accept, as full payment, minus applicable cost sharing)

- Invalid dates of service

- Missing or invalid modifiers

- Missing or invalid provider information, such as tax identification number

- Incorrect place of service

Other, less common possibilities include the following.

- Missing some tests and procedures

- Diagnosis and procedure coding errors or omissions

- Past filing limits for submission of claims

- Denial because the medical necessity provision has not been met

Managing Denials

It is important to track denials when payments are posted. Denials should be tracked by payer, type of denial, and provider. In a large medical practice, staff members should be assigned to work on denials on a daily basis.

If the reasons for denials start to look like a trend, providers or staff members should be informed. Then processes should be put in place to avoid the denials in the future. By addressing the denials as they come in, processes can be corrected on a timely basis.

It is best to avoid denials altogether. As a way to prevent them, staff members should be assigned to monitor correspondence, instructions, and other updates from high-volume payers. Information should be shared with the appropriate providers and staff members so claims can be completed and transmitted according to the payers' specifications.

---

medical necessity. The documented need for a particular medical intervention.

Denial Codes

Although the reasons for claim rejections are often similar, the way they are indicated on a claim varies from payer to payer. As an example of the kind of denial information sent to providers, it is useful to look at the system used by Medicare. Medicare uses nonmedical codes that provide more information about a claim, including why it was rejected.

These codes tend to fall into the following four categories.

- Group codes identify the party financially responsible for a specific service or the general category of payment adjustment.

- Claims adjustment reason codes (CARCs) provide financial information about claims decisions. Any payment adjustment must be accompanied by claims adjustment reason codes.

- Remittance advice remark codes (RARCs) further explain the reason for a payment adjustment. They are used with claims adjustment reason codes.

- Provider-level adjustment reason codes are not related to a specific claim. These adjustments are made by the provider's office.

The following tables show how these code adjustments might look like on a returned claim.

TABLE 4.2 *Group Codes*

CODE	PAYMENT ADJUSTMENT CATEGORY
CO	Contractual obligation: Used when a contractual agreement resulted in an adjustment. The provider is not allowed to bill the patient for the amount of the adjustment.
CR	Correction and renewal: Used for correcting a prior claim.
OA	Other adjustment: Used when no other code applies to the adjustment.
PR	Patient responsibility: Used to indicate the amount the patient owes, typically for deductible and coinsurance amounts.

TABLE 4.3 *Sample Codes Used for CARCs*

CODE	FINANCIAL INFORMATION
1	Deductible amount
2	Coinsurance amount
3	Copayment amount
4	The procedure code is inconsistent with the modifier used or the required modifier is missing.
5	The procedure code/bill type is inconsistent with the place of service.
40	Charges do not meet qualifications for emergent/urgent care.
96	Noncovered charge

TABLE 4.4 *Sample Codes used for RARCs*

CODE	MESSAGE
M1	X-ray not taken within the past 12 months or near enough to the time of treatment.
M2	Not paid separately when the patient is an inpatient.
M3	Equipment is the same or similar to equipment already being used.
M4	Alert: This is the latest monthly installment for a piece of equipment being used.
M125	Missing/incomplete/invalid information on the period of time that the supply/service/equipment will be needed.
N1	Alert: You may appeal this decision in writing after receiving this notice.
N24	Missing/incomplete/invalid electronic fund transfer.

TABLE 4.5 *Sample Provider-Level Adjustment Codes*

CODE	DEFINITION	USE
50	Late charge	Used to identify late claim filing penalty or Medicare late cost report penalty.
51	Interest penalty charge	Used to identify the interest assessment for late filing.
72	Authorized return	Used to identify a refund adjustment to an institutional provider from a previous overpayment.
90	Early payment allowance	Used to indicate when this has occurred.

Appeals Process

The Affordable Care Act (ACA) spells out how patients can appeal health insurance decisions. The following section explains what information the health insurance plan is required to send, how to request an internal appeal, and when to request an external independent review.

Information from the Insurance Company

The following information must be provided.

- The reason the claim was denied.

- An acknowledgment of the right of the patient to file an internal appeal.

- An acknowledgment of the right of the patient to request an external review if the internal appeal was unsuccessful.

- Identification of whether a Consumer Assistance Program is available. This will vary from state to state.

Requesting an Internal Appeal

After requesting an internal appeal, the plan must respond:

- 72 hours after receiving the request when the appeal is for a denial of a claim for urgent care. If the appeal concerns urgent care, it might be possible to have the internal appeal and external review take place at the same time.

- Within 30 days for denials of nonurgent care not yet received.

- Within 60 days for denials of services already received.

Requesting an External Independent Review

If the claim is still denied after the internal appeal, then a patient can request an external independent review. The plan must provide information on how to do this.

If the external independent review overturns the internal appeal process, then the insurer is required to pay for the claim.

Name two reasons why a claim may be denied.

ANSWER: An invalid subscriber name was given or a coding error was made.

SUMMARY

This chapter has covered the following points.

- What the revenue cycle is and how to document each part of it.

- How accounts receivable develops and manages aging reports.

- How to read a remittance advice.

- How to post payments.

- How to interpret denial codes.

- The steps of the appeals process.

The next chapter focuses on coding. Codes are documentation of the medical services patients receive. They are used by third-party payers to determine reimbursement for health care services. Understanding how to use codes properly when filling out claims is essential to the work of a billing and coding professional.

CHAPTER 4 DRILL QUESTIONS

Analyzing Aging Reports

1. What is the role of the accounts receivable department?

2. What are two kinds of information the CDM stores?

3. An aging report refers to which of the following?

    a. The length of time the report has been in the CDM

    b. The ages of all patients in a provider's practice

    c. The claims that are outstanding

    d. The amount of money the provider's office has received in the last 6 months

Interpreting Remittance Advice

4. True or False: An RA is sent to policyholders.

5. The allowable charge is which of the following?

    a. Amount the provider charges for a service

    b. Amount the patient agrees to pay

    c. Amount the health insurance company will pay providers

    d. Amount set by hospitals

Posting Payments

6. Which of the following is NOT a charge the patient is expected to pay?

    a. Coinsurance

    b. Deductible

    c. Difference between a provider's charges and what the insurance company will pay

    d. Copayment

7. The term reconciliation means which of the following?

    a. Resolving difference with the insurance company

    b. Working with Medicare on a problem

    c. Getting more information about a patient from a physician

    d. Determining how much the provider has been reimbursed and how much patients owe

Determining Reasons for Insurance Company Denial

8. What are the four types of nonmedical codes used by Medicare to explain claims?

9. Who benefits from the new appeals process, and why?

10. When can a patient request an external independent review?

CHAPTER 4 DRILL ANSWERS

1. The accounts receivable department manages follow-up to the billing process for a provider's office.

2. Among the correct responses are description of service, CPT/HCPCS code, revenue code, charge amount, charge or service code, general ledger key, and activity/status date.

3. **A.** *Incorrect* Aging reports do not include the length of time a report has been in the CDM.

   B. *Incorrect* Aging reports do not include ages of patients in a provider's office.

   C. *Correct* Aging reports refer to the paid or unpaid status of invoices.

   D. *Incorrect* Aging reports do not include the amount of money a provider's office has received in a specific time period.

4. False. An RA is sent to the provider, not to policyholders.

5. **A.** *Incorrect* The actual charge, also called the billed amount, refers to the amount the provider charges for the health care service.

   B. *Incorrect* The patient pays the provider usually in the form of deductibles and copayments.

   C. *Correct* The allowable charge, also called allowable fee, maximum fee, maximum allowable, usual-reasonable-customary, UCR charge, or prevailing rate, is the amount the insurer will actually pay.

   D. *Incorrect* Allowable charges are determined by insurance companies, not hospitals.

6. **A.** *Incorrect* The patient is expected to pay coinsurance.

   B. *Incorrect* The patient is expected to pay a deductible.

   C. *Correct* Write-offs are the amount a provider agrees to accept as payment minus deductibles, copayments, and coinsurance.

   D. *Incorrect* The patient is expected to pay a copayment.

7. **A.** *Incorrect* Reconciliation does not involve resolve differences with an insurance company.

   B. *Incorrect* Medicare patients receive a Medicare Summary Notice that explain how the third-party payer insurer determined the payment the provider will receive and the balance the policyholder must pay.

   C. *Incorrect* The RA, EOB, and MSN contain information needed to post payments to the appropriate parties. The provider's office uses these documents as a guide.

   D. *Correct* Reconciliation refers to the process the billing office goes through to determine what payments have come in from the third-party payer and what the patient owes the provider. The billing office uses the RA, EOB, and MSN to make these determinations.

8. Group codes, claims adjustment reason codes (CARCs), remittance advice remark codes (RARCs), and provider-level adjustment reason codes are not related to a specific claim. These adjustments are made by the provider's office.

9. The patient benefits because the new process lays out steps the insurance company must follow and makes sure that the tasks get done in a timely fashion.

10. The patient can request an external independent review after an internal appeal has been denied.

CHAPTER 5

Apply Knowledge of Coding

OVERVIEW

Chapters 1 through 4 of this study guide emphasized the importance of coding. Different kinds of codes are used for different purposes. Clinical coding systems, such as the International Classification of Diseases, Tenth Revision, Clinical Modification (ICD-10-CM), track a patient's diagnosis and clinical history. Procedural coding systems, such as Current Procedural Terminology (CPT) codes and the Healthcare Common Procedure Coding System (HCPCS), are used to report physician services for the purpose of reimbursement. The codes reported on claims are based on solid documentation, which has been discussed throughout this study guide.

This chapter presents an overview of the coding systems that billing professionals use. These include ICD-10-CM codes, CPT codes and modifiers, and HCPCS Level II codes. The chapter will explain the structure of ICD-10-CM, CPT, and HCPCS Level II codes. The chapter also discusses abstracting and coding from abstracted information.

Finally, this chapter provides a targeted overview of need-to-know medical terminology, functions of body systems, and types of health care facilities and providers.

By the end of this chapter, you should be able to answer the following questions.

1. List three purposes of ICD-10-CM.
2. True or False: The following represents a disease coded under ICD-10-CM: E10.2.
3. What are the goals of ICD-10-PCS?
4. What character of ICD-10 PCS for medical or surgical procedure would identify the body part?
   a. Character 1
   b. Character 2
   c. Character 3
   d. Character 4
5. CPT codes are used to describe which of the following?
   a. Supplies used during surgery
   b. Type of insurance a patient has
   c. Services rendered by the provider
   d. Payments received from third-party payers
6. What is the purpose for using modifiers?
7. What are HCPCS Level II codes used for?
8. Abstracting involves which of the following?
   a. Writing notes about codes
   b. Selecting relevant information from the health record
   c. Coding physicians' notes
   d. Answering questions from insurance companies
9. Abstracted information is which of the following?
   a. Sent to the physician
   b. Sent to the patient
   c. Coded
   d. Sent to the insurance company

CODING GUIDELINES AND CONVENTIONS FOR DIAGNOSES AND PROCEDURES

There are several kinds of coding systems. This section will focus on ICD-10-CM. Beginning on October 1, 2015, the U.S. switched to ICD-10-CM. This system is the standard for reporting diagnoses in all U.S. health care settings. The coding system serves as a way for health care professionals to let third-party payers, such as insurance companies or Medicare, know what diagnoses were treated. The system helps ensure that health care professionals and facilities are reimbursed in a timely manner.

The ICD coding and classification system is used worldwide. It is maintained by the World Health Organization (WHO), which updates it about every 10 years. The version being used internationally is ICD-10. The United States decided that ICD-10 needed to be modified before acceptance. The result is the system called ICD-10-CM/PCS. ICD-10-CM was developed by the Centers for Disease Control and Prevention (CDC) and is used in all U.S. health care settings. The International Classification of Diseases, 10th edition, Procedure Coding System (ICD-10-PCS) was developed by the Centers for Medicare and Medicaid Services (CMS) and is used only in U.S. hospital settings.

Using the ICD-10-CM Coding System

The ICD-10-CM/PCS coding system has separate manuals for diagnoses and procedures. Procedures are coded from the ICD-10-PCS manual, and diagnoses are coded from the ICD-10-CM manual. The ICD-10-PCS manual is discussed later. The designated uses of the ICD-10-CM system include the following.

- Classifying morbidity (number of cases of disease in a specific population) and mortality (incidence of death in a specific population)
- Indexing hospital records by disease and operations
- Reporting diagnoses by physicians
- Storing and retrieving data
- Reporting national morbidity and mortality data
- Serving as the basis of diagnosis-related group (DRG) assignment for inpatient hospital reimbursement
- Reporting and compiling health care data to assist in the evaluation of medical care planning for health care delivery systems
- Determining patterns of care among providers
- Analyzing payments for health services
- Conducting epidemiological and clinical research

Features of the ICD-10-CM

ICD-10-CM provides a high level of detail for diagnostic coding, which increases the accuracy of reporting codes for reimbursement, administrative, and statistical purposes. Features of the ICD-10-CM coding manual include the following.

- Provides more detailed clinical information, resulting in the following
  - Ability to measure health care services, such as the addition of information relevant to ambulatory and managed care encounters
  - Detailed injury and external cause codes
  - Sensitivity when refining grouping and reimbursement methodologies
  - Ability to conduct public health surveillance
  - Combination codes that reduce the number of codes needed to fully describe a condition
  - Decreased need to include supporting documentation with claims
- Current medical terminology and classification of diseases
- Codes that allow comparison of mortality and morbidity
- Data for the following
  - Measuring care given to patients
  - Designing payment systems
  - Processing claims
  - Making clinical decisions
  - Tracking public health
  - Identifying fraud and abuse
  - Conducting research

Structure of ICD-10-CM Codes and Manual

Code Structure

The code structure of ICD-10-CM consists of categories, subcategories, and codes. Each character for all categories, subcategories, and codes can be either a letter or number. Codes can be from three to seven characters in length. Only certain categories require the seventh character and sometimes placeholders (the letter x), as they are not required for all categories.

Three-Character Categories

Categories are three characters. Categories describe a single disease or condition, which is typically expanded by adding more characters (and more detail). The first category character is a letter; the second and third characters can be a number or letter. Each chapter begins with a list of three-character categories, such as A00-A09 Intestinal Infectious Diseases. ICD-10-CM refers to each of these grouped categories as blocks of codes.

Four-Character Sub-Categories

Codes that contain four characters provide definition for the site, the etiology and the manifestation or state of the disease or condition. For example, category C18 is malignant neoplasm of the colon. Reviewing the tabular list for this category demonstrates that the fourth character specifies greater detail for the site of the neoplasm.

Example:

C18 Malignant neoplasm of colon

> C18.**0** Malignant neoplasm of **cecum**
>
> C18.**1** Malignant neoplasm of **appendix**
>
> C18.**2** Malignant neoplasm of **ascending colon**
>
> C18.**3** Malignant neoplasm of **hepatic flexure**
>
> C18.**4** Malignant neoplasm of **transverse colon**
>
> C18.**5** Malignant neoplasm of **splenic flexure**
>
> C18.**6** Malignant neoplasm of **descending colon**
>
> C18.**7** Malignant neoplasm of **sigmoid colon**
>
> C18.**8** Malignant neoplasm of **overlapping sites of colon**
>
> C18.**9** Malignant neoplasm of colon, **unspecified**

Five-Six Character Classification

Codes that contain a fifth or sixth character provide the greatest level of specificity in the code set. For example, code M13.11 describes Monoarthritis, not elsewhere classified, of the shoulder. The sixth character indicates laterality of the Monoarthritis.

Example:

M13.11 Monoarthritis, not elsewhere classified, shoulder

> M13.11**1** Monoarthritis, not elsewhere classified, **right shoulder**
>
> M13.11**2** Monoarthritis, not elsewhere classified, **left shoulder**
>
> M13.11**9** Monoarthritis, not elsewhere classified, **unspecified shoulder**

Placeholders

Codes that require a seventh character extension don't always contain six characters. The missing character(s) are filled in with a placeholder (the letter X) until the seventh character extension can be placed. For example, the code for a foreign body in the right ear is represented by code T16.1. This code requires a seventh character extension. Since the code is only four characters in length, placeholders are needed for the fifth and sixth characters. Then the required seventh character can be applied.

Example:

T16.1**XX**A Foreign body in right ear, initial encounter

Seventh Character Extension

Certain categories require a seventh character extension, typically in the injury and fracture categories. If a category indicates the need for a seventh character, it must be applied and must remain in the seventh character position. The tabular list will provide guidance for applicable seventh character extensions.

The seventh character typically identifies the episode of care (initial, subsequent, or sequela). In applicable fracture categories, it also identifies the type of fracture (open, closed, or type) and the healing phase of the patient (routine, delayed, nonunion, or malunion).

Example:

S62.241 Displaced fracture of shaft of first metacarpal bone, right hand

S62.241**A** ...... **initial encounter for closed fracture**

S62.241**B** ...... **initial encounter for open fracture**

S62.241**D** ...... **subsequent encounter for fracture with routine healing**

S62.241**G** ...... **subsequent encounter for fracture with delayed healing**

S62.241**K** ...... **subsequent encounter for fracture with nonunion**

S62.241**P** ...... **subsequent encounter for fracture with malunion**

S62.241**S** ...... **sequela**

Manual Structure

The ICD-10-CM coding manual can be arranged according to the wishes of its various publishers. It is, however, typically similar in content. The main components of an ICD-10-CM manual are:

- Preface/Introduction
- Official ICD-10-CM Conventions and Guidelines
- Alphabetic Index to Diseases
- Neoplasm Table
- Table of Drugs and Chemicals
- Index to External Causes
- Tabular List of Diseases and Injuries
  - 21 chapters of codes, arranged according to body system or disease process
- Appendixes

Some manuals contain additional resources such as anatomy plates, and instructions to correct coding. Familiarizing yourself with the details and resources of your manual is important to improving speed and accuracy in coding.

Coding Guidelines and Conventions for Diagnoses and Procedures

Each ICD-10-CM and ICD-10-PCS coding manual requires the use of coding conventions and contain official coding guidelines for correct code assignment. While essential reading for use of both coding manuals, these guidelines are critical for correct code assignment and sequencing instructions for ICD-10-CM and ICD-10-PCS.

Conventions and General Coding Guidelines include:

- Abbreviations
  - NEC "Not elsewhere classifiable" An alphabetic index entry that states NEC directs the coder to an "other specified" code in the Tabular List.
  - NOS "Not otherwise specified" This abbreviation is the equivalent of "unspecified."
- Use of "And" and "With"
  - The word "and" should be interpreted to mean either "and" or "or" when it appears in a title.
  - The word "with" or "in" should be interpreted to mean "associated with" or "due to" when it appears in a code title, the Alphabetic Index, or an instructional note in the Tabular List.
- Excludes Notes
  - Excludes1 indicates the code excluded should never be used at the same time as the code above the Excludes1 note. The exception is when the provider documents that both conditions exist, and more than one code is assigned.
  - Excludes2 indicates the condition excluded is not part of the condition represented by the code, but from a patient who may have both conditions at the same time. Thus, the assignment of multiple codes are permitted.
- Code First/Use Additional Code Notes
  - Etiology/manifestation paired codes have specific sequencing
    - The etiology code first
    - The manifestation code (in brackets) sequenced second; do not enter the brackets when reporting manifestation codes
- Locating a code: Read and be guided by instructional notations that appear in both the Index and the Tabular List.
- Level of detail in coding: A code is invalid if it has not been coded to the full number of characters required for that code.
- Signs and Symptoms: should not be reported with a confirmed diagnosis if the symptom is integral to the diagnosis.
- Multiple coding for a single condition: conditions that require more than one code. The notation "Code, if applicable, any causal condition first," will be referenced.
- Acute and Chronic Conditions: If the same condition is described as acute and chronic, and separate subentries exist in the alphabetic index
  - Code both, and sequence the acute condition first.

- Combination Code: a single code used to classify
  - Two diagnoses, or a diagnosis with an associated secondary process (e.g., manifestation)
  - A diagnosis with an associated complication

- Late Effects (Sequela): the residual effect (condition produced) after the acute phase of an illness or injury has terminated.

- Impending or Threatened Condition: If the condition did occur, code as a confirmed diagnosis. If it did not occur, reference the alphabetic index to determine if the condition has a subentry term for impending or threatened. If the subterms are listed, assign the subterms. If they are not listed, code the existing underlying conditions or signs/symptoms.

- Documentation of Complications of Care: a cause-and-effect relationship between the care provided and the condition, and an indication in the documentation that it is a complication.

Basic Features and Format of ICD-10-PCS Coding System

ICD-10-PCS codes are made up of seven digits using numbers and 24 letters (A-H, J-N, and P-Z) The letters are not case-sensitive, and letters O and I are not used to avoid confusion with numbers zero and one. No decimal points are used. Procedures are divided into 16 sections related to whether it is a medical, surgical, imaging, or other kind of procedure. All procedure codes have seven characters. The first digit always corresponds to the section where the procedure is classified. The second through seventh characters have specific meanings, which are identified below.

EXAMPLE OF MEDICAL/SURGICAL SECTION CHARACTER MEANINGS

1 = Section of the ICD-10-PCS system where the code is indexed

2 = The body system

3 = Root operation, such as excision or incision

4 = Specific body part

5 = Approach used

6 = Device used to perform the procedure

7 = Qualifier to provide additional information about the procedure (diagnostic vs. therapeutic)

EXAMPLE OF AN ICD-10-PCS CODE AND HOW TO INTERPRET IT

Code: 097F7DZ

Section: Medical and surgical 0

Body system: Ear, nose, sinus 9

Root operation: Dilation 7

Body part: Eustachian tube, right F

Approach: Via natural or artificial opening 7

Device: Intraluminal (done with tubes) D

Qualifier: No qualifier Z

HEALTHCARE COMMON PROCEDURE CODING SYSTEM (HCPCS)

HCPCS is a group of codes and descriptors used to represent health care procedures, supplies, products, and services. HCPCS is divided into two levels: I and II. Level I is the Current Procedure Terminology (CPT-4) codes, which are maintained by the American Medical Association. Level II codes, also called National Codes, are maintained by the Centers for Medicare and Medicaid (CMS). Each of these levels is described in the next sections.

CPT HCPCS Level I

CPT is a uniform code that accurately describes and reports medical, surgical, and diagnostic services and procedures. Physicians use CPT codes for hospital inpatient and outpatient services and for those performed in other facilities. Because the CPT code set was adapted for Medicare, it is referred to as HCPCS Level I in the coding and reimbursement communities.

CPT Code Categories

CPT codes are divided into Category I, II, and III groupings.

Category I CPT codes are five-digit codes and two-digit modifiers. Modifiers use both Level I and Level II HCPCS to change the code description. For example, modifier 50 is used to describe a bilateral procedure. Modifier 52 indicates that a procedure was decreased or limited.

Category I CPT codes primarily cover physicians' services but are used for hospital outpatient coding, too. Category I sections and codes are listed below. Each of these sections has guidelines with specific instructions and definitions. The CPT manual is composed of six chapters, referred to as sections. The sections are further divided into subsections, subheadings, categories, and subcategories.

To code correctly, coders must understand the information in the guidelines.

- Evaluation and Management   99201-99499
- Anesthesia   00100-01999, 99100-99140
- Surgery   10021-69990
- Radiology   70010-79999
- Pathology and Laboratory   80047-89398
- Medicine (excluding Anesthesia)   90281-99199, 99500-99607

According to the AMA, ***Category II*** codes were designed to serve as supplemental tracking codes that can be used for performance measurement. Although these codes are optional, they do help provide more information about a patient's visit and treatment plan.

Category III codes are used for temporary coding for new technology and services that have not met the requirements needed to be added to the main section of the CPT book. These codes are not optional. They should be used to report procedures performed.

Codes in this section are evaluated and added every 6 months. As Category I codes are created to describe new procedures, the temporary Category III codes are deleted. If Category III codes are not used after about 5 years, they are deleted.

Appendixes

Appendixes are in the last section of codes. They provide information to the coder. The following sections describe each appendix and what they contain.

- **APPENDIX A** has a complete list of modifiers and their descriptions. Modifiers are written as two-digit codes that follow the main CPT codes.

- **APPENDIX B** is a summary of the additions, deletions, and revisions that have been put into use in the current CPT edition. This information can help the coder make sure that he is using the most current information.

- **APPENDIX C** has clinical examples for codes in the evaluation and management section of the CPT book. They are helpful in understanding how to report a code in this section.

- **APPENDIX D** is a listing of CPT add-on codes. These codes must be preceded by a primary procedure code. They should never be reported alone.

- **APPENDIX E** is a summary of CPT codes that are exempt from modifier 51.

- **APPENDIX F** is a summary of CPT codes exempt from modifier 63.

- **APPENDIX G** has codes that include conscious/moderate sedation but was removed from CPT.

- **APPENDIX H** is an alphabetic index of performance measures by clinical conditions or type but was removed from CPT.

- **APPENDIX I** has genetic testing code modifiers used for reporting with lab procedures related to genetic testing but was removed from CPT.

- **APPENDIX J** includes a list of sensory, motor, and mixed nerves that are useful for nerve conduction studies.

- **APPENDIX K** lists procedures included in the CPT codebook that are not yet approved by the FDA.

- **APPENDIX L** is a reference of the vascular families, including which are considered first-, second-, and third-order vessels.

- **APPENDIX M** shows a table of deleted CPT codes and crosswalks to current codes.

- **APPENDIX N** is a listing of codes that have been resequenced.

- **APPENDIX O** lists multianalyte assays with algorithmic analyses and proprietary laboratory analyses.

- **APPENDIX P** lists CPT codes that can be used for synchronous telemedicine services.

Category I CPT code. Code that covers physicians' services and hospital outpatient coding.

Category II CPT code. Code designed to serve as supplemental tracking codes that can be used for performance measurement.

Category III CPT code. Code used for temporary coding for new technology and services that have not met the requirements needed to be added to the main section of the CPT book.

Index

The CPT codebook index lists main terms in alphabetical order. Main terms include the following six ways to locate a procedure, also referred to as the Location Method.

- Procedure or service

- Just anatomic site

- Condition or disease

- Synonym, eponym, or abbreviation

Subterms follow main terms. Subterms modify the main terms and are indented under them. To search for the correct CPT code, coders check the alphabetic index in the order listed above until finding a code to describe the procedure performed. The coder should then look in the code section of the codebook to validate that this is the appropriate code selection or assignment.

Management of CPT

The AMA's CPT Editorial Panel is responsible for revising the CPT codebook, which takes place once a year. The panel gets advice from the CPT Advisory Committee. This committee is nominated by the AMA House of Delegates and is made up of representatives from more than 90 medical specialty societies and other health care professional organizations.

The CPT Advisory Committee is charged with meeting the following three objectives.

1. To serve as a resource to the editorial panel by giving advice on procedure coding and nomenclature as relevant to the member's specialty.

2. To provide documentation to staff and the editorial panel regarding the medical appropriateness of various medical and surgical procedures.

3. To suggest revisions to CPT.

HCPCS Level II

HCPCS Level II codes were established to report services, supplies, and procedures not represented in CPT. These codes begin with a letter from A-V, followed by four numbers. The letter identifies the code section and type of service or supply. Descriptions identify items or services, not specific brand names. Table 5.2 lists the code categories for HCPCS Level II.

TABLE 5.2 *HCPCS Level II Code Categories*

CATEGORIES	WHAT THEY COVER	INSURERS
A codes	Ambulance and transportation services, medical and surgical supplies, administrative, miscellaneous, and investigational services and supplies	All payers
B codes	Enteral and parenteral therapy	All payers
D codes	Dental	All payers
E codes	Durable medical equipment	All payers
G codes	Procedures/professional services (temporary)	
J codes	Drugs that are usually not self-administered, such as chemotherapy, immunosuppressive drugs, and inhalation solutions	All payers
L codes	Orthotic and prosthetic procedures and devices	All payers
M codes	Office services and cardiovascular and other medical services	All payers
P codes	Pathology and laboratory services	All payers
Q codes	Temporary codes	
R codes	Domestic radiology services	All payers
V codes	Vision, hearing, and speech-language pathology services	All payers

HCPCS Level II Modifiers

HCPCS also allows for modifiers, which can be used for all levels of HCPCS codes, including CPT codes. They add more specific information to what's referenced in the main code. Table 5.3 shows some examples of HCPCS Level II modifiers.

TABLE 5.3 *Examples of HCPCS Level II Modifiers*

CODE	WHAT IT STANDS FOR
AA	Anesthesia services performed personally by anesthesiologist
E1	Upper left eyelid
E2	Lower left eyelid
E3	Upper right eyelid
E4	Lower right eyelid
NU	New equipment
QC	Single channel monitoring

How many CPT code category sections are listed in the CPT manual?

ANSWER: Six CPT code category sections are listed in the CPT manual.

ABSTRACTING MEDICAL DOCUMENTATION

Transferring Information from Encounter Forms

An encounter is the term used to describe a direct, professional visit between a patient and a health care professional, such as a physician, who is licensed to provide medical services, including diagnosis and treatment. During the encounter, physicians document in the health record information about past history, current history, inpatient admissions, and hospital discharge information. This information is used for claim submission and the reimbursement process. Sometimes it is used for research and clinical quality performance reviews.

It is the role of the coder to abstract information from the encounter form and other sources. Abstracting involves reviewing the health record and encounter form for code assignment and entering it into a computer database. Below is a sample of the kind of information that needs to be abstracted and put into a computer database. A coder can have as many as 200 data items from each record to abstract.

FIGURE 5.1 *Sample Encounter Form*

Patient Encounter Form		*Family Health Practice*
Patient Information	**Payment Method**	**Visit Information**
Patient ID #	Primary	Date
Patient name	Primary ID #	Physician
Address	Primary group #	Referral
City/State	Secondary	Reason for visit
Contact #	Secondary ID #	
DOB/Age	Secondary group #	

Office Visits		**Procedures**		**Diagnosis - ICD-10-CM**	
New Patient		81002	Urine, dip	Abd pain, unspec	R10.9
99201	Minimal office visit	82948	Glucose, blood stick	Anemia, unspec	D64.9
99202	20 min	85018	Hemoglobin	Bronchitis, unspec	J20.9
99203	30 min	99173	Visual acuity	Burn	T30.0
99204	45 min	92551	Hearing screening	Conjunctivitis	H10.13
99205	60 min	36415	Venipuncture	Contact dermatitis	L25.9
Established Patient		36416	Finger stick	Contusion	T14.9
99211	Minimal office visit	86580	PPD	Cough	R05
99212	20 min	46600	Anoscopy	Dental caries	K02.9
99213	30 min	**Immunizations**		Disorders of teeth	K08.9
99214	45 min	90471	IZ Admin # 1	Enuresis	F98.0
99215	60 min	90472	IZ Admin # 2	Foreign body, eye	T15.9
Preventive Medicine Visits		90472	IZ Admin # 3	Foreign body, soft tis.	M79.5
New Patient		90472	IZ Admin # 4	Headache, unspc	R51
99381	Less than 1 year	90472	IZ Admin # 5	Hearing problem	R68.8
99382	1 to 4 years	90713	IPV	Hygiene	Z72.9
99383	5 to 11 years	90700	DTaP	General exam, normal	Z00.00
99384	12 to 17 years	90648	HIB	General exam, abnormal	Z00.01
99385	18 to 39 years	90633	Hepatitis A	Immunization	Z23
99386	40 to 64 years	90744	Hepatitis B	Impacted cerumen	H61.23
99387	65+ years	90707	MMR	Impetigo	L01.0
Established Patient		90716	Varicella	Injury to eye	S05.9
99391	Less than 1 year	90658	Influenza	Injury, superficial	T07.0
99392	1 to 4 years			Lice, head	B85.0
99393	5 to 11 years			Medication dispensed	Z76.0
99394	12 to 17 years			Nausea & vomiting	R11.2
99395	18 to 39 years			Otitis media, acute	H66.009
99396	40 to 64 years			OM w/ rupture of TM	H66.019
99397	65+ years			Pharyngitis	J02.9
				PPD screen	Z11.1
Vitals		**Other Visit Information**		School exam	Z02.89
BP		Lab orders		Splinter, finger	S60.45
Pulse				Tonsillitis, acute	J03.90
Temp				URI, acute, NOS	J06.9
Height		Notes		UTI, unspec	N39.0
Weight				Vision problem	H54.7

Follow up with provider? ☐ Yes ☐ No
Follow-up date:
Further treatment plan:

Signature:
Date:

RANDI HARDY
ASSESSMENT TECHNOLOGIES INSTITUTE

encounter form. Form that includes information about past history, current history, inpatient record, discharge information, and insurance information.

abstracting. The extraction of specific data from a medical record, often for use in an external database, such as a cancer registry.

The information below in Table 5.4 is provided by the hospital admissions department and discharge planning department.

TABLE 5.4 *Information to Extract from an Encounter Form*

ADMIT SOURCE	INPATIENTS/OUTPATIENTS	ASA CLASSIFICATION
Against medical advice	Skilled nursing inpatients	Gestation
Physician referral	Surgical inpatients	C-section
Psychiatric facility	Oncology inpatients	No previous C-section
Clinic referral	Obstetrics	Previous C-section
HMO referral	Trauma	C-section performed for complications
Long-term care facility	Newborn	VBAC (vaginal birth after C-section)
Transfer from a hospital	Cardiology	
Intermediate care facility	Medicine	
Transfer from another health care facility	**DISCHARGE FACILITY**	**TRANSFER FACILITY**
Assisted living	Anesthesia type	Hospital service
Emergency room	Conscious sedation	Hospice inpatient
Hospice	General	Psychiatric and alcohol
Court/law enforcement	Monitored anesthesia care	
Home health	Regional	
Information not available	**DISCHARGE DISPOSITION**	**BIRTH WEIGHT**
	Self-care (home)	Acute care facility
	Skilled nursing facility	Expired
	Rehabilitation facility	Unknown
		APGAR SCORE (0-10)

Source: Health Information Managment Techonlogy: An Applied Approach, pg. 394/ Adapted from materials provided by OhioHealth, Columbus, OH

---

encoder. Software that suggests codes based on documentation or other input.

MS-DRG grouper. Software that helps coders assign the appropriate Medicare severity diagnosis-related group based on the level of services provided, severity of the illness or injury, and other factors.

APC grouper. Helps coders determine the appropriate ambulatory payment classification (APC) for an outpatient encounter.

---

computer-assisted coding (CAC). Software that scans the entire patient's electronic record and codes the encounter based on the documentation in the record.

Coding Abstracted Information

It is also the role of the billing and coding profession to assign the correct code. This process is abstracting, which involves translating diagnostic and procedural information into the correct code, such as ICD-10-CM, CPT, and HCPCS Level II. This can be done manually or by using a computer program called an encoder. This program helps guide the coder through the abstracting process and assists with inputting the correct diagnosis, procedural, or service code.

Another part of the encoding system for acute care hospitals is called MS-DRG software that leads the coder to the appropriate MS-DRG by sorting out the medical documentation the coder inputs. This role requires the coder to review the documentation with great detail before entering information into the software. APC groupers help coders determine the appropriate ambulatory payment classification for an outpatient encounter.

FIGURE 5.2 *Encoder Example*

Code	Description
10021	fine needle aspir; w/o image guide
10022	fine needle aspir; w/ image guide
10060	i&d of abscess; simple or single
10061	i&d of abscess; complicated / multi
10080	i&d of pilonidal cyst; simple
10081	i&d of pilonidal cyst; complicated

RANDI JANELL HARDY
ASSESSMENT TECHNOLOGIES INSTITUTE

As more health care facilities move to an electronic environment, computer-assisted coding (CAC) may be used to generate the correct codes for each episode of care. However, the codes assigned by the CAC software must be checked by a medical coding professional for accuracy.

Coding can be done periodically or at the time of discharge from care. When the coding is done periodically, the coding professional checks the health record every few days and puts in the appropriate codes. Coding done at the time of discharge means that the professional will have to include all the diagnoses, procedures, and services the patient experienced during the hospital stay.

Consulting with Physicians

Because accurate documentation is so important, the billing and coding professional should go over the abstracted documents and/or coding information form with the physician if he or she has any questions about the notes on the form. Also, if the staff member is unsure how to abstract or code a specific item, she should consult with the physician before moving forward. Because reimbursement depends on correct coding, it's always better to be "safe rather than sorry."

What is abstracting?

ANSWER: Abstracting involves reviewing the health record and/or encounter form and translating the medical documentation into the specific code sets. The code set data is then entered into the computer database.

COMMON MEDICAL TERMINOLOGY

Terms based on anatomy used to describe diagnoses and procedures are referred to as medical terminology. These terms can be broken down into four basic word parts.

1. Root (primary word origin)

2. Combining form (root word + vowel, usually an o or sometimes i) to connect the word group to make it complete for easier pronunciation

3. Prefix (word group at the beginning of the term)

4. Suffix (word group at the end of the term).

Without a thorough knowledge of medical terms, it is impossible to correctly perform billing and coding functions. However, once you master the basic parts, most medical terms can be understood, even if you are seeing it for the first time.

TABLE 5.5 *Combining Forms*

ROOT WORD + VOWEL	MEANING
nephr/o	kidney
gastr/o	stomach
col/o	colon, large intestines
cardi/o	heart
my/o	muscle
mamm/o	breast
cyst/o	pelvis
pelv/o	bladder
crani/o	cranium (skull)
erythr/o	red

FIGURE 5.3 *Anatomical Directional Terms*

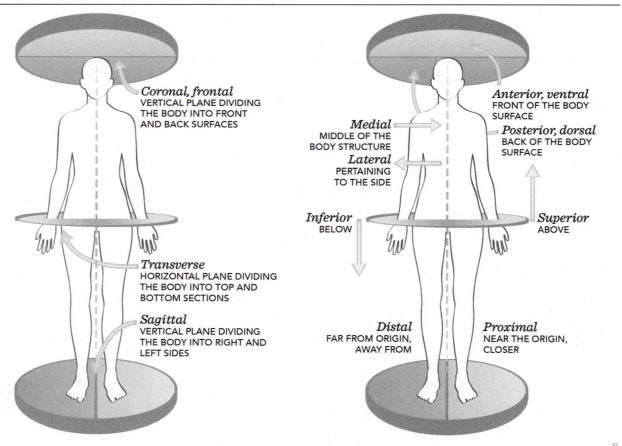

Coronal, frontal
VERTICAL PLANE DIVIDING THE BODY INTO FRONT AND BACK SURFACES

Transverse
HORIZONTAL PLANE DIVIDING THE BODY INTO TOP AND BOTTOM SECTIONS

Sagittal
VERTICAL PLANE DIVIDING THE BODY INTO RIGHT AND LEFT SIDES

Medial
MIDDLE OF THE BODY STRUCTURE

Lateral
PERTAINING TO THE SIDE

Anterior, ventral
FRONT OF THE BODY SURFACE

Posterior, dorsal
BACK OF THE BODY SURFACE

Inferior
BELOW

Superior
ABOVE

Distal
FAR FROM ORIGIN, AWAY FROM

Proximal
NEAR THE ORIGIN, CLOSER

TABLE 5.6 *Common Medical Prefixes, Suffixes, and Root Words*

DIAGNOSTIC SUFFIXES	MEANING	PROCEDURAL SUFFIXES	MEANING
-algia	pain	-centesis	surgical puncture
-emia	blood condition	-ectomy	removal, resection, excision
-itis	inflammation	-gram	record
-megaly	enlargement	-graphy	process of recording
-meter	measure	-lysis	separation, breakdown, destruction
-oma	tumor, mass	-pexy	surgical fixation
-osis	abnormal condition	-plasty	surgical repair
-pathy	disease condition	-rrhaphy	suture
-rrhagia	bursting forth of blood	-scopy	visual examination
-rrhea	discharge, flow	-stomy	opening
-sclerosis	hardening	-therapy	treatment
-scopy	to view	-tomy	incision, to cut into

PREFIXES	MEANING	ROOT WORDS	MEANING
a-, an-	without	arth	joint
ante-	before	cephal	head
anti-	against	cholecyst	gall bladder
brady-	slow	chondro	cartilage
dys-	painful, difficult	colp	vagina
endo-	inside, within	derm	skin
epi-	upon, above	enter	intestine
ex-	out, out of	episi	vulva
hemi -	half, partial	gastro	stomach
hypo-	below, deficient	gloss	tongue
infra-	below	hepato	liver
inter-	between	hyster	uterus
neo-	new	lapar	abdomen
pan-	all	lact	milk
para-	beside	lith	stone
per-	through	mast	breast
poly-	many	myo	muscle
pre-	before, in front of	nat	birth
pseudo-	false	oophor	ovary

Body Systems and Their Functions

To assign the correct procedure and diagnosis codes to a medical claim, you must understand the human body and its directional terms in order to comprehend provider reports and other medical documentation. The human body consists of body systems, each of which is designed to fulfill a different function.

The digestive system is responsible for ingesting and digesting food, absorbing nutrients, and eliminating waste. The main organs of the digestive system include the mouth, tongue, salivary glands, pharynx, esophagus, stomach, small intestine, large intestine (colon), rectum, anus, pancreas, liver, and gallbladder.

The respiratory system is responsible for delivering oxygenated blood to all parts of the body. Through breathing, the body inhales oxygen and exhales carbon dioxide, warms and moisturizes the air, and filters debris. The main organs of the respiratory system include the pharynx, larynx, nasal cavity, oral cavity, trachea, lungs, bronchus, bronchioles, and alveoli.

The musculoskeletal system gives the human body form and stability and enables movement. It consists of bones, muscles, tendons, ligaments, joints, cartilage, and other connective tissue. Connective tissue is made of elastic fibers and collagen, a protein substance. Connective tissue assists in the support function of the musculoskeletal system. Providers that specialize in treating patients who have musculoskeletal injuries or illnesses are physiatrists, specialists in physical medicine and rehabilitation, or orthopedic surgeons.

The integumentary system regulates body temperature, acts as a sensory receptor to internal and external stimuli, excretes waste from the body through sweat, and absorbs vitamin D and calcium from sunlight to nourish the body. The major parts of the integumentary system include the epidermis, dermis, and hypodermis or subcutaneous layers, sebaceous glands, sudoriferous glands, pores, reticular layer, and melanin.

The cardiovascular system delivers nutrients and oxygen to every cell within the body and removes waste products. The major organs of the cardiovascular system are the heart and blood vessels, known as arteries and veins. The heart muscle is comprised of three layers: the endocardium (inner layer), myocardium (middle layer), and pericardium (outer layer). The pericardium is a double-walled sac that encloses the heart. Infectious micro-organisms, cancerous growths, and other problems can cause the pericardium to be inflamed, called pericarditis. The endocardium forms the lining of the heart. Endocarditis is the condition that results when infectious micro-organisms enter the endocardium. The infection can then spread to further affect the valves of the heart. The myocardium is the thickest layer of the heart. With each heartbeat, the muscle fibers contract and squeeze the blood. Myocarditis is an inflammation of the heart. Cardiomyopathy literally means heart muscle disease and is a generalized diagnosis of primary heart disease. The coronary arteries are blood vessels that supply oxygen directly to the heart tissue. A myocardial infarction (MI), or heart attack, is caused by a lack of oxygen and results in heart damage. Sometimes MIs can be caused by coronary heart disease, which occurs when there is a narrowing of the small blood vessels that supply oxygen to the heart muscle.

The circulatory and lymphatic systems are responsible for the overall balance of body system functions. These systems involve the fluids of the body. The circulatory system provides cells within the body with nutrients, while the lymphatic system rids the body of unnecessary substances. Oxygen-rich blood is transported to all parts of the body via arteries. The blood travels through arterioles and then into the vessels with the thinnest walls, known as capillaries. The thin walls allow for the exchange of oxygen, nutrients to the cells, and waste from the cells. Oxygen and carbon dioxide also are exchanged within the capillaries. The blood flows from the capillaries back to the heart through the venules. From there, the blood flows into the veins. This process repeats itself when the veins carry the blood back to the heart. In the heart, the pulmonary vein carries blood to the lungs where carbon dioxide is exchanged for oxygen.

The lymphatic system and the circulatory system are closely related structures joined by the capillary system. The lymphatic system distributes fluids and nutrients throughout the body and drains excess fluids and protein to prevent edema. Edema is the retention of excess fluids in the body. This fluid is referred to as lymph and contains white blood cells, proteins, and fats. Lymph seeps outside the blood vessels and is stored in the lymphatic system to flow back into the bloodstream. The flow of blood in and out of the blood vessels and through the lymph nodes enables the body to eliminate waste products and excess fluid.

The urinary system aids in the process of secreting and eliminating urine. The urinary system includes the urethra, bladder, ureters, and kidneys. These organs produce, collect, and eliminate urine. Ureters are the route by which urine exits the kidneys and connects to the bladder, where urine is stored until it is expelled via the urethra. The process of excretion is the elimination of wastes from the body. Wastes are eliminated in multiple ways. For example, the respiratory system eliminates carbon dioxide, the digestive system removes solid waste, and skin eliminates toxins through perspiration. Urination, or the act of excreting urine, occurs when our bodies produce waste from metabolizing the foods we eat. The elimination of waste by the kidneys is imperative to maintaining good health. The reduced ability of the kidneys to perform their necessary functions is called renal insufficiency, while renal failure is the complete failure of kidney function. Diffusing blood to remove toxins and maintain balance is called dialysis. Hemodialysis is necessary when the kidneys fail to remove wastes from the bloodstream. Diuretics are liquids that increase the process of urination. The most common diuretics are water, coffee, and tea. Polyuria is a term that means excessive urination.

The endocrine system is a system of glands that produces and secretes hormones. Hormones regulate the body's growth, metabolism, sexual development, and function. These hormones release into the bloodstream and act as chemical messengers in the body. The major glands of the endocrine system include the hypothalamus, pituitary, thyroid, parathyroids, adrenals, pineal body, and the reproductive organs (ovaries and testes). The pancreas, which produces hormones and aids in digestion, is also part of the system.

The nervous system consists of the central nervous system (CNS) and the peripheral nervous system (PNS). It receives information and interprets it via electrical signals carried by the nerves. The CNS is divided into two parts: the brain and the spinal cord. The spinal cord conducts sensory information from the peripheral nervous system to the brain and information from the brain to the skeletal muscles, cardiac muscle, smooth muscle, and glands. The brain receives sensory input from the spinal cord, as well as from its own nerves. The PNS's main function is to connect the CNS to the limbs and organs. It is divided into the sensory nervous system and the motor nervous system.

The reproductive system is the system by which humans reproduce. The organs of the female reproductive system include the ovaries, fallopian tubes, uterus, vagina, and mammary glands. The male reproductive system includes the testes, scrotum, penis, vas deferens, and prostate.

HOSPITAL TERMINOLOGY

Types of Facilities

Health care facilities are identified by the type of facility and services they provide. For example, what is commonly referred to as a **hospital** is typically a short-term acute care facility, or general hospital. Other health care facilities include **psychiatric hospitals**, **rehabilitation facilities**, **clinics**, **nursing homes**, **subacute hospitals**, and **home health care agencies**. Inpatient facilities are equipped for patients to stay overnight. In addition to hospitals, inpatient care is also provided at skilled nursing facilities and long-term care facilities. Services that do not require an overnight stay are referred to as outpatient care, also called ambulatory care.

Hospital Departments

In a general hospital system, there are many departments. Each of these departments is designed to address specific health care needs.

The department of pediatrics is responsible for meeting the medical needs of infants, children, and teenagers. In contrast, the department of internal/family medicine is responsible for meeting the needs of patients of all ages and addressing a wide range of patient health concerns. However, both these departments treat a variety of medical issues.

The department of internal/family medicine refers the patient to a specialty department for further treatment she needs more advanced screening and care.

The department of urology, a specialty department, treats patients for illnesses or conditions related to the urinary system. Urologists are physicians who specialize in the study or practice of urology, which is the study of conditions related to the urinary tract.

The department of dermatology, a specialty department, treats patients who have medical conditions that affect the integumentary system, or skin, hair, and nails. This department sees patients whose skin conditions range from mild, such as dermatitis or acne, to severe, such as burns or skin cancer.

The department of cardiology or the department of cardiovascular medicine is a specialty department that is responsible for the treatment of patients who have medical illnesses or conditions related to the heart and vascular system. Patients might have heart disease, angina, congestive heart failure (CHF), arrhythmias, or heart murmurs.

The department of pathology specializes in the study of disease. For example, when the department receives a biopsy of skin or tissue, a pathologist carefully examines the specimen to detect changes in cell structure, color, texture, or growth. The result of gross and microscopic examination assists pathologists in determining the behavior or morphology of the cells. Patients can be diagnosed with malignant (cancerous) or benign (non-cancerous) tumors. The pathologist then reports the findings to the requesting provider for further treatment recommendations.

Laboratory Testing

The pathology and laboratory departments are often combined in hospital settings. The laboratory is responsible for processing blood, body fluid, and tissue specimens from patients and performing a variety of analytical tests or examinations requested by a licensed medical professional.

The procedure for obtaining samples of blood is called venipuncture. A patient's blood is usually drawn to detect levels of normal and abnormal chemicals in the bloodstream, such as potassium, or the amount of white or red blood cells.

Another laboratory procedure is a urinalysis (UA). A urinalysis is a group of tests performed on a urine sample. A common UA is performed to detect excess bacteria in urine. Excess bacteria can cause urinary tract infections (UTIs) and bladder infections. A UA can also be used to detect pregnancy. Blood tests can also be ordered for the purpose of detecting pregnancy. Combinations of laboratory tests are often used to diagnose specific issues. For example, to evaluate kidney function, a combination of a blood test and a UA can be used. The blood, urea, and nitrogen (BUN) blood test can be used along with a creatinine urine test to help diagnose kidney disease.

Identifying Health Care Providers

The departments within a hospital are composed of professional clinical and administrative staff. Clinical staff is involved in direct medical patient care, while administrative staff supports patient care.

Attending or staff physicians are generally more experienced than most other physicians, primarily because they have completed their residency and fellowship requirements. After assessing a patient, resident and fellow physicians consult with a staff physician before rendering a final diagnosis. The staff physician is responsible for diagnosing conditions in patients, performing procedures necessary to treat patients, and for directing any follow-up care or referrals necessary to promote a healthy prognosis for patients. Staff physicians complete at least 8 years of clinical/hospital education and training. Attending or staff physicians have final responsibility, both legal and otherwise, for the care of patients admitted to the hospital. Attending or staff physicians issue orders for patients. These include written, telephone, fax, or consultation orders for new or altered treatment. The orders are then carried out by the clinical staff, including nurses and medical assistants. Orders can consist of administering medication, obtaining vital signs, immobilizing the patient after surgical procedures, or dietary restrictions.

Referring physicians refer patients for services or supplies that they cannot directly provide. They direct patients to other hospital departments or specialists for treatment. Many health maintenance organizations (HMOs) require patients to have referral from their primary care physicians (PCP) before seeking specialist care. The idea is to ensure the lowest-cost, highest-quality care by making sure all specialist visits are medically necessary. If a PCP deems it necessary for a patient to be referred to another provider, then a visit to a specialist is granted by the health care plan, and the cost of the visit or procedure is billable to and paid by the health plan. However, if a patient who has an HMO insurance plan is seen by a specialist without receiving a referral from his PCP, then the health plan does not reimburse the provider for services.

Resident physicians have finished medical school and their internship and are currently receiving training in a specialized area. They have completed a medical clerkship program and successfully completed their U.S. Medical Licensing Examination to meet the educational requirements for entrance into a residency training program. Fellow physicians enter a training program in a medical specialty after completing residency, typically in a hospital or academic setting.

Registered nurses (RNs) are graduate nurses who have been legally authorized (registered) to practice after passing an examination given by a state board of nurse examiners or similar regulatory authority. RNs work closely with providers and other professionals in the health care setting. Their position is unique because they act as a liaison between the patient, provider, medical assistant, and often the medical coding and billing specialist. They are responsible for carrying out verbal and written orders, such as administering vaccinations and medications, monitoring a patient's vital signs, performing blood draws and laboratory tests, and assisting with procedures, such as Papanicolaou (Pap) tests, suture removal, and invasive and non-invasive surgical procedures. RNs obtain an Associate of Science, Bachelor of Science, or Master of Science degree in nursing.

Licensed practical nurses (LPNs) are able to perform functions similar to an RN, but under the direct supervision of an RN. For example, LPNs are trained to collect various samples for laboratory testing and perform routine laboratory tests. According to the Department of Labor, in some states, LPNs are permitted to administer prescribed medicines, start intravenous fluids, and provide care to ventilator-dependent patients. LPNs can work in hospitals or other specialized settings, such as nursing homes, providers' offices, or home health care. To become an LPN, there is a minimum of 12 months of medical training required.

Medical assistants (MAs) are also an integral part of the health care system. Like nurses, they work closely with providers, patients, administrative staff, and other health care professionals. Medical assistants perform administrative and clinical tasks to keep providers' offices running smoothly. They also can perform some basic functions of medical billing and coding. Although they are not required to, medical assistants can complete certification examinations, such as the Certified Clinical Medical Assistant (CCMA) or the Certified Medical Assistant (CMA) examination. Depending on the program, it can take 9 to 24 months of specialized training to become a medical assistant.

Medical administrative assistants are responsible for providing administrative support to health care providers and other health care professionals. Medical administrative assistants perform general office tasks, such as answering telephones, greeting patients, handling correspondence, scheduling appointments, making travel arrangements, registering patients for their visits, and maintaining the patient schedule. Like medical assistants, medical administrative assistants are also able to perform basic billing and coding functions. Formerly, medical administrative assistants were known as secretaries and receptionists. However, their titles have changed, as the duties and responsibilities of these positions have increased. Although certification is not required, those who obtain formal training and become a certified medical administrative assistant receive higher pay, advance into higher positions, and are recognized by their peers as highly qualified in their field.

Medical coding and billing specialists hold an important role in the health care setting. They are responsible for obtaining the maximum reimbursement for providers for all services rendered. They make sure that clean, error-free claims are submitted to insurance carriers in a timely manner. You are required to appropriately complete and submit medical insurance claims, and have a thorough understanding of insurance carriers and their specific procedures, including government, private, and commercial companies. Furthermore, you should demonstrate a thorough knowledge of coding systems, coding guidelines and convention, medical terminology, and anatomy and physiology.

SUMMARY

This chapter has covered the following topics.

- The purpose of coding

- The structure of ICD-10-CM

- The structure of CPT and HCPCS Level II codes

- How to use these code

- Abstracting information

- Coding after the abstraction process is completed

- Medical terminology

- Body systems and their functions

- Types of health care facilities and providers

The five chapters in this study guide have discussed many topics of importance to billing and coding professionals: the importance of keeping compliant with official guidelines, how to prepare and process claims, how to read documents from third-party payers and use them to post payments accurately, and how to abstract information from the health medical record and code it correctly.

Understanding these concepts and how they are related are important for billing and coding professionals. This study guide has illustrated those connections and provided information needed for aspiring billing and coding professionals to become accredited in the field.

CHAPTER 5 DRILL QUESTIONS

Coding Guidelines and Conventions for Diagnoses and Procedures

1. List three purposes of ICD-10-CM.

2. True or False: The following represents a disease coded under ICD-10-CM: E10.2.

3. What are the goals of ICD-10-PCS?

4. What character of ICD-10 PCS for medical or surgical procedure would identify the Medical/Surgical section's body part?

    a. Character 1

    b. Character 2

    c. Character 3

    d. Character 4

Healthcare Common Procedure Coding Systems (HCPCS)

5. CPT codes are used to describe which of the following?

    a. Supplies used during surgery

    b. Type of insurance a patient has

    c. Services rendered by the provider

    d. Payments received from third-party payers

6. What is the purpose for using modifiers?

7. What are HCPCS Level II codes used for?

Abstracting Medical Documentation

8. Abstracting involves which of the following?

    a. Writing notes about codes

    b. Selecting relevant information from the health record

    c. Coding physicians' notes

    d. Answering questions from insurance companies

9. Abstracted information is which of the following?

    a. Sent to the physician

    b. Sent to the patient

    c. Coded

    d. Sent to the insurance company

CHAPTER 5 DRILL ANSWERS

1. Among the correct responses are classifying morbidity and mortality, indexing hospital records by disease and operations, reporting diagnoses by physicians, storing and retrieving data, reporting national morbidity and mortality data, serving as the basis of diagnosis-related group assignment for hospital reimbursement, reporting and compiling health care data, determining patterns of care among providers, analyzing payments for health services, and conducting epidemiological and clinical research.

2. True. For ICD-10-CM codes, the first character is a letter, followed by digits. Characters three through seven can be numbers or letters.

3. The goals of ICD-10-PCS are to improve accuracy and efficiency of coding, reduce training effort, and improve communication with physicians.

4. **A.** *Incorrect* Character 1 identifies the site.
   B. *Incorrect* Character 2 identifies the body system.
   C. *Incorrect* Character 3 identifies the root operation.
   D. *Correct* Character 4 identifies the body part.

5. **A.** *Incorrect* HCPCS codes describe supplies used during surgery.
   B. *Incorrect* CPT codes provide information for insurance companies, not about insurance companies.
   C. *Correct* Physicians use CPT codes for hospital inpatient and outpatient services and for those performed in other facilities.
   D. *Incorrect* The ICD-10-CM system is used to analyze payments for health services.

6. Modifiers provide the means to report or indicate a service or procedure that has been altered by some specific circumstance but not changed in its definition or code.

7. HCPCS Level II codes were established to report services, supplies, and procedures not represented in CPT.

8. **A.** *Incorrect* Billing and coding professionals interpret notes about codes, but this is not abstracting.
   B. *Correct* Abstracting involves reviewing the health record and or encounter form and translating the medical documentation into the specific code sets.
   C. *Incorrect* Physicians' notes are not coded, but interpreting physicians' notes are part of coding.
   D. *Incorrect* Abstracting does not include questions from insurance companies.

9. **A.** *Incorrect* Abstracted information is not sent to the physician.
   B. *Incorrect* Abstracted information is not sent to the patient.
   C. *Correct* Abstracted information is coded, often using computer-assisted coding to generate codes for each episode of care.
   D. *Incorrect* Abstracted information is not sent to the insurance company.

IN PRACTICE
Case Studies

CASE STUDY 1: DETERMINING PATIENT COVERAGE

Dr. Martin stops Mary, the billing and coding specialist, in the hallway of the provider's office.

"Hi, Mary," he says. "I need you to research a case for me. Suzy Smith is one of my patients. I'm considering a manipulation under anesthesia, but I'd like to be sure her insurance will cover the procedure."

Mary smiles and says, "No problem, Dr. Martin. I'll look into it and get back to you."

QUESTION 1 *What information does Mary need to begin her research?*

Mary needs to verify the patient's identity, including the patient's age. She also needs to verify the patient's insurance coverage information and eligibility.

QUESTION 2 *What clinical information does Mary need to obtain?*

Mary needs to obtain the exact procedure Dr. Martin will be performing in order to determine the correct CPT code. She also needs to obtain the preoperative diagnosis (or diagnoses) Dr. Martin will be using to determine the correct ICD-10-CM diagnosis code(s). If Mary is unfamiliar with any of the medical terms, she will need to consult a medical dictionary or another reliable source for definitions. In addition, she should consult with the provider if further clinical information is needed to determine coding.

QUESTION 3 *What steps should Mary take to ensure the procedure will be covered?*

Mary should research the insurance carrier's policy concerning the procedure. Medical policy information can include age restrictions, policy exclusions, and a listing of diagnosis code(s) the insurance carrier will accept to justify medical necessity for the procedure. Mary should also obtain preauthorization from the insurance carrier to ensure the procedure is medically necessary and covered.

QUESTION 4 *What should Mary do if the insurance carrier's policy does not allow the procedure with the diagnosis code(s) Dr. Martin wishes to use?*

Mary should speak with the provider to verify the diagnosis. Mary must be careful to avoid leading the provider toward the insurance carrier's diagnosis code selection. It is unethical and can be considered insurance fraud for a billing and coding specialist to lead a provider in code selection for the sole purpose of obtaining reimbursement.

QUESTION 5 *In addition to coverage, what information should Mary obtain from the insurance carrier before reporting her findings to Dr. Martin?*

Mary should determine if preauthorization is required by the insurance carrier for the procedure. If preauthorization is required, Mary should obtain a preauthorization number from the insurance carrier for the procedure. It might be necessary for Mary to obtain the scheduled date of surgery before the insurance carrier issues a preauthorization.

QUESTION 6 *How will Mary determine the portion of any covered amount that may be the patient's responsibility?*

Mary will research the patient's benefits and policy restrictions through the insurance carrier. Mary may also obtain predetermination from the insurance carrier to confirm the maximum dollar amount that the insurance carrier will pay for the procedure and any patient responsibility.

CASE STUDY 2: BILLING MISTAKE

A patient, Donna Shipley, calls Patrick, a certified billing and coding specialist, saying she received a bill for medical treatment she did not receive. The 72-year-old patient has an explanation of benefits for $191 for a prenatal visit on October 1.

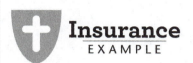

Insurance
E X A M P L E

P.O.BOX 99999
Anywhere, USA 12345
Customer Service 1.800.555.1234

Donna Shipley
123 Main Street
Anywhere, USA 12345

EXPLANATION OF BENEFITS
This is not a bill.

Enrollee:	Shipley, Donna
Patient ID #:	BBB00000
Provider:	Eleanor Richardson, OB/GYN
Claim #:	111111111111111
Date Processed:	11/07/2014

Dates of Service	Description of Service	CPT Code	Charge Amount	Allowed Amount	Not Covered	Co-Pay	Benefit Amount	Due from Patient
10/1/2014	prenatal visit	99213	$110.00		$110.00			$110.00
10/1/2014	incision and removal - complicated	10121-22	$59.00		$59.00			$59.00
10/1/2014	lab draw	36415	$15.00		$15.00			$15.00
10/1/2014	general health panel	80050	$7.00		$7.00			$7.00

Total Due from Patient
$191.00

RJH
ASSESSMENT TECHNOLOGIES INSTITUTE

Patrick looks up the patient's name, and there are two Donna Shipleys in the system. One had a prenatal visit on October 1, and one had a postoperative appointment on the same day.

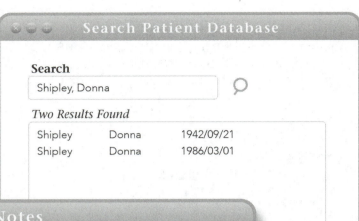

Search Patient Database

Search

Shipley, Donna

Two Results Found

| Shipley | Donna | 1942/09/21 |
| Shipley | Donna | 1986/03/01 |

Progress Notes

Name:	Shipley, Donna	**Date of Service:**	1 Oct 2014
ID #:	BBB111111111	**DOB:**	21 Sep 1942
Provider:		**Gender:**	Female

| **Description:** | Postoperative Care |

Procedures	**CPT Code**
Incision and removal - complicated	10121-22
Lab draw	36415
General health panel	80050

Subjective

Patient came into office today complaining of painful cyst on left forearm that has been there for 5 days. Patient also here today to receive lab work for physical exam already scheduled.

Ob...

Progress Notes

Name:	Shipley, Donna	**Date of Service:**	1 Oct 2014
ID #:	BBB000000000	**DOB:**	1 Mar 1986
Provider:	Richardson, Eleanor	**Gender:**	Female

| **Description:** | Prenatal Visit |

| **Procedures** | **CPT Code** |
| Prenatal visit | 99213 |

Subjective

Patient returns for 2 week prenatal visit. She has no complaints today.

Objective

All vital signs are stable. BP 119/80 P 75 Weight 140. No reports of elevated BP or edema. The fetus heart rate is strong and active moment is reported at time of visit. Uterine size about 2 cm measuring on target.

RJH
ASSESSMENT TECHNOLOGIES INSTITUTE

QUESTION 1 *What steps should Patrick take to resolve this inquiry?*

Patrick should retrieve both Donna Shipley accounts, verify charges submitted, review progress notes to determine which patient receive which services, and contact the insurance company to see how they want this claim corrected. (Each payer has a different process for corrected claims.) Once the correct coding has been identified and selected, a corrected claim for the correct Donna Shipley should be resubmitted to the carrier, and the patient should be contacted to inform that the account has been resolved.

QUESTION 2 *What information needs to be collected from the patient to verify identity?*

Patrick will need the patient's full name, date of birth (DOB), copy of insurance card front and back, and a copy of the patient's ID.

QUESTION 3 *What could have been done to prevent this error?*

Patrick could have prevented this error by not identifying the member by name only. When entering charges, the patient's name, DOB, and insurance must always be verified in addition to reviewing all selected items on the superbill before entry.

QUESTION 4 *What part of the EOB identifies which procedure was not received by the client?*

Patrick can identify the procedures not received by the client on the EOB by viewing the description of service and CPT code listed.

QUESTION 5 *What steps need to happen to identify the correct patient ID number?*

Patrick needs to get a front-and-back copy of the patient's ID card. Then this information needs to be validated against what was submitted on the claim and what was entered into the practice management system.

CASE STUDY 3: DENIED INSURANCE FORM

A certified coding and billing specialist, John, receives a confusing superbill from a provider. John deciphers them as best as he can and submits the claim to the client's insurance company.

The insurance claim is denied because the information is inaccurate. John must figure out what's wrong with the form and resubmit.

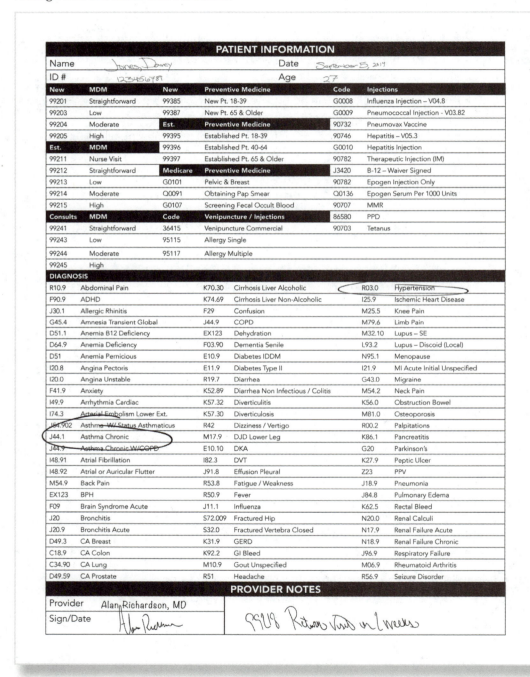

John goes back to the superbill and follows up with the provider on the correct CPT of 99213 and not 99218. The provider pulls the record, reviews the progress notes, and sees that the code was illegible.

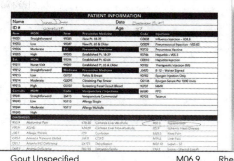

| | M10.9 | Gout Unspecified | M06.9 | Rheumato... |
| | R51 | Headache | R56.9 | Seizure Diso... |

PROVIDER NOTES

n, MD

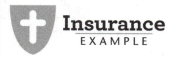

Insurance
EXAMPLE

Davey Jones
987 Main Street
Anywhere, USA 12345

EXPLANATION OF BENEFITS

Enrollee:	Jones, Davey
Patient ID #:	BBB123456789
Provider:	Alan Richardson, MD
Claim #:	777777777777
Date Processed:	11/07/2014

Dates of Service	Description of Service	CPT Code	Charge Amount	Allowed Amount	Not Covered	Co-Pay	Benefit Amount	Due from Patient
9/5/2014	Predetermination	99218	$150.00		$150.00			$150.00

Total Due from Patient
$150.00

Progress Notes

Name:	Jones, Davey	**Date of Service:**	5 Sep 2014
ID #:	BBB123456789	**DOB:**	21 Sep 1987
Provider:	Alan Richardson, MD	**Gender:**	Male

Description: knee pain, hypertension

Procedures	CPT Code
E&M level 3, evaluation management	99213

Subjective

Patient came into the office presented with knee pain. Patient had expanded problem with hypertension for 14 days.

Objective

Mr. Jones is here to f/u on hypertension and to discuss the onset of his knee pain. Weight 280, pulse 78, BP 160/90. A possible trigger to the expanded hypertension is poor exercise and obesity. No known accidents or previous injuries.

QUESTION 1 *What was the identifier in the SOAP note to determine which level of service should be billed?*

John can identify the level of service in the progress note by reviewing the documentation of history place of service, type of service, and patient status. The documentation varies depending on the complexity of the services provided and the specialty of the physician.

QUESTION 2 *What should John have done after receiving the superbill?*

John should have reviewed the superbill completely. The CPT code entered was for observation services. John should know that, based on the location and type of service, the code selection was invalid and should have been questioned. In addition, if a CBCS is ever confused, he should check with the provider before submitting the claim.

QUESTION 3 *How can illegible superbills be prevented?*

To prevent illegibly written superbills, the provider should adopt an EMR system or complete the form by circling or checking off the correct CPT code and instead of hand-writing it. A CBCS can assist by returning all incomplete and unchecked/uncircled superbills to the provider.

QUESTION 4 *What is the importance of the provider having legible documentation?*

The provider having legible documentation avoids denials or delays in payments when clinical information is requested. If records are ever subpoenaed, legible records can hold up in court. Legible documentation enforces compliance.

QUESTION 5 *How was the provider able to determine the correct procedure billed?*

The provider was able to determine the CPT code by retrieving the superbill to decipher what was written, and then validating the correct CPT based on clinical documentation written in the progress note.

QUESTION 6 *What should John do prior to resubmitting the claim to the insurance company?*

This is no longer a resubmitting claim; it is a corrected claim. John should contact the insurance for the process to submit a corrected claim to prevent the claim from being denied as a duplicate submission of same date service, location, and provider. Resubmitting the claim with the correct code only will not guarantee payment.

APPENDIX
References

Casto, A. B., and Forrestal, E. (2013). *Principles of healthcare reimbursement* (4th Ed.). Chicago, IL: AHIMA Press. pp. 75.

Centers for Medicare & Medicaid Services. (April 2013). *ICD-10-CM/PCS: The next generation of coding.* Retrieved June 17, 2014, from https://www.cms.gov/Medicare/Coding/ICD10/downloads/ICD-10Overview.pdf

Centers for Medicare & Medicaid Services. (November 27, 2013). *Physician self referral.* Retrieved June 17, 2014, from http://www.cms.gov/Medicare/Fraud-and-Abuse/PhysicianSelfReferral/

Centers for Medicare & Medicaid Services. (October 2010). *Understanding the remittance advice: A guide for Medicare providers, Physicians, Suppliers, and Billers.* Retrieved June 17, 2014, from http://www.cms.gov/Outreach-and-Education/Medicare-Learning-Network-MLN/MLNProducts/downloads/ra_guide_full_03-22-06.pdf

Centers for Medicare & Medicaid Services. (Rev. December 27, 2013). *Medicare claims processing manual.* Chapter 26. Retrieved from June 17, 2014, from http://www.cms.gov/Regulations-and-Guidance/Guidance/Manuals/downloads/clm104c26.pdf

Centers for Medicare & Medicaid Services. (Rev. January 25, 2013). *Important information regarding the Centers for Medicare & Medicaid Services (CMS) national claims crossover process.* Retrieved from June 17, 2014, from http://www.cms.gov/Outreach-and-Education/Medicare-Learning-Network-MLN/MLNMattersArticles/downloads/SE0909.pdf

Claim adjustment reason codes: ASC X12 external code source 139. (April 23, 2014). Washington Publishing Company. Retrieved June 17, 2014, from http://www.wpc-edi.com/reference/codelists/healthcare/claim-adjustment-reason-codes

Crocker, Janice. (October 2006). *How to improve your revenue cycle processes in a clinic or physician practice.* AHIMA's 78th National Convention and Exhibit Proceedings. Retrieved June 17, 2014, from http://library.ahima.org/xpedio/groups/public/documents/ahima/bok1_035391.hcsp?dDocName=bok1_035391

Federal Trade Commission. (November 2013). *Debt collection.* Retrieved June 17, 2014, from https://www.consumer.ftc.gov/articles/0149-debt-collection

Insure.com. (August 3, 2012). *"Birthday rule" determines health insurance coverage.* Retrieved June 17, 2014, from http://www.insure.com/articles/healthinsurance/birthday-rule.html

Medical Billing and Coding Online. *Medical billing insurance claims process.* Retrieved June 17, 2014, from http://www.medicalbillingandcodingonline.com/medical-billing-claims-process/

New York State Department of Health. (February 2010). *Medicare crossover process frequently asked questions.* Retrieved June 17, 2014, from https://www.emedny.org/medicare_crossover/medicare_crossover_faqs.pdf

Polisky, Robert A. (May/June 2013). *How the new HIPAA regulations affect billing companies and their subcontractors as business associates: Develop an action plan for your company and subcontractors.* HBMA Billing. Retrieved June 17, 2014, from http://www.hbma.org/news/public-news/n_how-the-new-hipaa-regulations-affect-billing-companies-and-their-subcontractors-as-business-associates

Reimbursement Concepts University. *The insurance verification process.* Retrieved June 17, 2014, from http://www.rcuonline.net/images/InsuranceVerificationProcess.pdf

Sayles, Nanette B. (Ed.) (2013). *Health information management technology: An applied approach* (4th ed.). Chicago: American Health Information Management Association.

U.S. Department of Health & Human Services, Agency for Healthcare Research and Quality. *AHRQ quality indicators toolkit.* Retrieved June 17, 2014, from http://www.ahrq.gov/professionals/systems/hospital/qitoolkit/b4-documentationcoding.pdf

U.S. Department of Health & Human Services. *Appealing health plan decisions.* Retrieved June 17, 2014, from http://www.hhs.gov/healthcare/rights/appeal/appealing-health-plan-decisions.html

U.S. Department of Health and Human Services, Center for Medicare & Medicaid Services. (November 2012). *Medicare fraud & abuse: Prevention, detection, and reporting.* Retrieved June 17, 2014, from http://www.cms.gov/Outreach-and-Education/Medicare-Learning-Network-MLN/MLNProducts/downloads/Fraud_and_Abuse.pdf

U.S. Department of Health and Human Services, Centers for Medicare & Medicaid Services. (August 2013). *Medicare enrollment and claim submission guidelines.* Retrieved June 17, 2014, from http://www.cms.gov/Outreach-and-Education/Medicare-Learning-Network-MLN/MLNProducts/downloads/MedicareClaimSubmissionGuidelines-ICN906764.pdf

APPENDIX
Glossary

A

abstracting. The extraction of specific data from a medical record, often for use in an external database, such as a cancer registry.

abuse. Practices that directly or indirectly result in unnecessary costs to the Medicare program.

account number. Number that identifies specific episode of care, date of service, or patient.

accounts receivable department. Department that keeps track of what third-party payers the provider is waiting to hear from and what patients are due to make a payment.

activity/status date. Indicates the most recent activity of an item.

actual charge. The amount the provider charges for the health care service.

Administration Simplification Compliance Act (ASCA). Specifically prohibits any payment by Medicare for services or medically necessary supplies that are not submitted electronically.

administrative services only (ASO) contract. Contract between employers and private insurers under which employers fund the plans themselves, and the private insurers administer the plans for the employers.

Advance Beneficiary Notice of Noncoverage. Form provided if a provider believes that a service may be declined because Medicare might consider it unnecessary.

aging report. Measures the outstanding balances in each account.

allowable charge. The amount an insurer will accept as full payment, minus applicable cost sharing.

APC grouper. Helps coders determine the appropriate ambulatory payment classification (APC) for an outpatient encounter.

assignment of benefits. Contract in which the provider directly bills the payer and accepts the allowable charge.

auditing. Review of claims for accuracy and completeness.

authorization. Permission granted by the patient or the patient's representative to release information for reasons other than treatment, payment, or health care operations.

B

balance billing. Billing patients for charges in excess of the Medicare fee schedule.

batch. A group of submitted claims.

Blue Cross and Blue Shield plan. The first prepaid plan in the U.S. that offers health insurance to individuals, small businesses, seniors, and large employer groups.

business associate (BA). Individuals, groups, or organizations who are not members of a covered entity's workforce that perform functions or activities on behalf of or for a covered entity.

C

capitation. The fixed amount a provider receives.

case management. A review of clinical services being performed.

Category I CPT code. Code that covers physicians' services and hospital outpatient coding.

Category II CPT code. Code designed to serve as supplemental tracking codes that can be used for performance measurement.

Category III CPT code. Code used for temporary coding for new technology and services that have not met the requirements needed to be added to the main section of the CPT book.

charge amount. The amount the facility charges for the procedure or service.

charge description master (CDM). Information about health care services that patients have received and financial transactions that have taken place.

charge or service code. Internally assigned number unique to each facility.

claim. A complete record of services provided by a health care professional, along with appropriate insurance information, submitted for reimbursement to a third-party payer.

claims adjustment reason code (CARC). Provides financial information about claims decisions.

claim scrubber. Software that reviews a claim prior to submission for correct and complete data, such as accurate gender in alignment with diagnosis/procedure or medical necessity.

clean claim. Claim that is accurate and complete. They have all the information needed for processing, which is done in a timely fashion.

clearinghouse. Agency that converts claims into a standardized electronic format, looks for errors, and formats them according to HIPAA and insurance standards.

clinical documentation. The record of clinical observations and care a patient receives at a health care facility.

commercial insurance. Private and employer-based self-insurance.

computer-assisted coding (CAC). Software that scans the entire patient's electronic record and codes the encounter based on the documentation in the record.

conditional payment. Medicare payment that is recovered after primary insurance pays.

consent. A patient's permission evidenced by signature.

contractual obligation. Used when a contractual agreement resulted in an adjustment.

coordination of benefits rules. Determines which insurance plan is primary and which is secondary.

correction and renewal. Used for correcting a prior claim.

cost sharing. The balance the policyholder must pay to the provider.

crossover claim. Claim submitted by people covered by a primary and secondary insurance plan.

D

de-identified information. Information that does not identify an individual because unique and personal characteristics have been removed.

demographic information. Date of birth, sex, marital status, address, telephone number, relationship to subscriber, and circumstances of condition.

description of service. An evaluation and management visit, observation, or emergency room visit.

diagnosis code. International Classification of Diseases (ICD-10-CM).

dirty claim. Claim that is inaccurate, incomplete, or contains other errors.

E

electronic data interchange (EDI). The transfer of electronic information in a standard format.

employer-based self-insurance. Insurance that is tied to an individual's place of employment.

encoder. Software that suggests codes based on documentation or other input.

encounter. A direct, professional meeting between a patient and a health care professional who is licensed to provide medical services.

encounter form. Form that includes information about past history, current history, inpatient record, discharge information, and insurance information.

explanation of benefits (EOB). Describes the services rendered, payment covered, and benefit limits and denials.

F

Fair Debt Collection Practices Act (FDCPA). Debt collectors cannot use unfair or abusive practices to collect payments.

False Claims Act. Protects the government from being overcharged for services provided or sold, or substandard goods or services.

Final Rule. Strengthens the HIPAA ruling around privacy, security, breach notification, and penalties.

formulary. A list of prescription drugs covered by an insurance plan.

fraud. Making false statements of representations of material facts to obtain some benefit or payment for which no entitlement would otherwise exist.

G

gatekeeper. Provider who determines the appropriateness of the health care service, level of health care professional called for, and setting for care.

general ledger key. Two- or three-digit number that makes sure that a line item is assigned to the general ledger in the hospital's accounting system.

group code. Code that identifies the party financially responsible for a specific service or the general category of payment adjustment.

group or plan number. Unique code used to identify a set of benefits of one group of type of plan.

group practice model. HMO that contracts with an outside medical group for services.

H

Health Insurance Portability and Accountability Act (HIPAA) of 1996. Legislation that includes Title II, the first parameters designed to protect the privacy and security of patient information.

health maintenance organization (HMO). Plan that allows patients to only go to physicians, other health care professionals, or hospitals on a list of approved providers, except in an emergency.

health record number. Number the provider uses to identify an individual patient's record.

I

ICD-10-CM. Coding and classification system that captures diseases and health-related conditions. Developed by the World Health Organization (WHO) and adapted to the U.S. health care system for uses that include securing reimbursement for services provided.

ICD-10-PCS. Coding and classification system developed for use in the U.S. only. Specific to inpatient hospital procedures.

implied consent. A patient presents for treatment, such as extending an arm to allow a venipuncture to be performed.

independent practice association (IPA) model. HMO that contracts with the IPA, which in turn contracts with individual health providers.

individually identifiable. Documents that identify the person or provide enough information so that the person could be identified.

informed consent. Providers explain medical or diagnostic procedures, surgical interventions, and the benefits and risks involved, giving patients an opportunity to ask questions before medical intervention is provided.

M

managed care organization. Organization developed to manage the quality of health care and control costs.

Medicaid. A government-based health insurance option that pays for medical assistance for individuals who have low incomes and limited financial resources. Funded at the state and national level. Administered at the state level.

medical necessity. The documented need for a particular medical intervention.

Medicare Administrative Contractor (MAC). Processes Medicare Parts A and B claims from hospitals, physicians, and other providers.

Medicare Advantage (MA). Combined package of benefits under Medicare Parts A and B that may offer extra coverage for services such as vision, hearing, dental, health and wellness, or prescription drug coverage.

Medicare. Federally funded health insurance provided to people age 65 or older, people younger than 65 who have certain disabilities, and people of all ages with end-stage kidney disease. Funded and administered at the national level.

Medicare Part A. Provides hospitalization insurance to eligible individuals.

Medicare Part B. Voluntary supplemental medical insurance to help pay for physicians' and other medical professionals' services, medical services, and medical-surgical supplies not covered by Medicare Part A.

Medicare Part D. A plan run by private insurance companies and other vendors approved by Medicare.

Medicare specialty plan. Plan that provides focused, specialized health care for specific groups of people, such as those who have both Medicare and Medicaid, live in a long-term care facility, or have chronic medical conditions.

Medicare Summary Notice (MSN). Document that outlines the amounts billed by the provider and what the patient must pay the provider.

Medigap. A private health insurance that pays for most of the charges not covered by Parts A and B.

modifier. Additional information about types of services, and part of valid CPT or HCPCS codes.

morbidity. The number of cases of disease in a specific population.

mortality. The incidence of death in a specific population.

MS-DRG grouper. Software that helps coders assign the appropriate Medicare severity diagnosis-related group based on the level of services provided, severity of the illness or injury, and other factors.

N

National Provider Identifier (NPI). Unique 10-digit code for providers required by HIPAA.

network model. HMO that contracts with two or more independent practices.

Notice of Exclusions from Medicare Benefits. Notification by the physician to a patient that a service will not be paid.

O

ordering provider. A physician or other licensed health care professional (e.g., physician assistant, nurse practitioner) who prescribes services for a patient.

other adjustment. Used when no other code applies to the adjustment.

out-of-network. Not contracted with the health plan.

out-of-pocket maximum. A predetermined amount after which the insurance company will pay 100% of the cost of medical services.

P

patient responsibility. The amount the patient owes.

preauthorization. The health plan is notified that a hospital stay or significant procedure is coming up, giving the plan the opportunity to determine if it is medically necessary and, in the case of an inpatient admission, how many days the patient most likely will need to stay.

precertification. A review that looks at whether the procedure could be performed safely but less expensively in an outpatient setting.

predetermination. A written request for a verification of benefits.

preferred provider organization (PPO). Plan that allows patients to use physicians, specialists, and hospitals in the plan's network.

preferred provider. Tier 2 provider.

primary insurance. Insurance that pays first, up to the limits of its coverage.

prior approval number. Number indicating that the insurance company has been notified and has approved services before they were rendered.

Privacy Rule. A HIPAA rule that establishes protections for the privacy of individual's health information.

private fee-for-service plan. Plan that allows patients to go to any physician, other health care professional, or hospital as long as the providers agree to treat those patients.

private insurance. Health care subsidized through premiums paid directly to the company.

procedure code. ICD procedure codes (ICD-10-PCS), Current Procedural Terminology (CPT) codes, or the Healthcare Common Procedures Coding System (HCPCS) that represents the procedure or service.

protected health information (PHI). Individually identifiable health information.

provider-level adjustment reason code. Codes that are not related to a specific claim.

R

referral. Written recommendation to a specialist.

referring provider. The physician or other licensed health care professional who requests a service for a patient.

reimbursement. Payment for services rendered from a third-party payer.

remittance advice (RA). The report sent from the third-party payer to the provider that reflects any changes made to the original billing.

remittance advice remark code (RARC). Code that explains the reason for a payment adjustment.

revenue code. Four-digit code that identifies specific accommodation, ancillary service, or billing calculation related to services on a bill.

S

staff model. HMO that provides hospitalization and physician services through its own staff.

Stark Law. Physicians are not allowed to refer patients to a practitioner with whom they have a financial relationship.

State Children's Health Insurance Program (SCHIP). A program jointly funded by the federal government and the states.

subscriber number. Unique code used to identify a subscriber's policy.

subscriber. Purchaser of the insurance or the member of group for which an employer or association as purchased insurance.

supervising provider. The physician monitoring a patient's care.

T

third-party payer. Organization other than a patient who pays for services, such as insurance companies, Medicare, and Medicaid.

Tier 1. Providers and facilities in a PPO's network.

Tier 2. Providers and facilities within a broader, contracted network of the insurance company.

Tier 3. Providers and facilities out of the network.

Tier 4. Providers and facilities not on the formulary.

timely filing requirement. Within 1 calendar year of a claim's date of service.

U

UB-04 code. Three-digit code that describes a classification of a product or service provided to the patient.

unbundling. Using multiple codes that describe different components of a treatment instead of using a single code that describes all steps of the procedure.

upcoding. Assigning a diagnosis or procedure code at a higher level than the documentation supports, such as coding bronchitis as pneumonia.

utilization review. A process used to determine the medical necessity of a particular procedure or service, designed to ensure that the procedure or service is appropriate and is being provided in the most cost-effective way.

W

write-off. The difference between the provider's actual charge and the allowable charge.

APPENDIX
Index

Figures and tables are indicated by "f" and "t" following page numbers.